365 SIMPLE PLEASURES

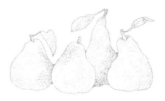

365 SIMPLE PLEASURES

collected by **Susannah Seton**

CONARI PRESS

Berkeley, California

Conari Press books are distributed by Publishers Group West.

Cover Photography: © Steve Cole/PhotoDisc
Cover and Book Design: Claudia Smelser
Interior Illustrations: Jonathan Robertson, Joan Carol

Library of Congress Cataloging-in-Publication Data

Seton, Susannah, 1952–
    365 simple pleasures : daily suggestions for comfort and joy / Susannah Seton.
        p.   cm.
    ISBN 1-57324-708-1
    1. Women—Conduct of life—Miscellanea. 2. Recipes.
    I. Title: Three hundred sixty-five simple pleasures. II. Title.
BJ1610 .S44 2001
646.7—dc21   2001002143

Printed in the United States of America on recycled paper.

01 02 03 04   RRD NW 10 9 8 7 6 5 4 3 2 1

We are not sent into this world to do anything into which we cannot put our hearts.

John Ruskin

FOREWORD

by Gail Greco

author of *Secrets of Entertaining* and *Tea-Time at the
Inn*, and host/producer of the award-winning PBS TV
series, *Country Inn Cooking with Gail Greco*

During the past twenty years, while I've been writing about bed-and-breakfast inns, innkeepers have led me not only through the doors of their charming, well-appointed, and thoughtful rooms and their delicious, homemade meals. In addition, surrounded by the great halo of their hospitality, I have learned about myself and about others. Once I asked an innkeeper, "So, what do you do on those days when you want to shut out the world, but in just a few short hours, guests will be arriving, seeking your undivided attention and whatever is left of your energy?"

On a high note, she challenged me, "Having a bad day? What a great time to invite someone over!"

What an incredible comment, I thought. But the she was right. As she had discovered—by having no choice in the matter—if she could pull herself up, suppress her doldrums, and muster up strength with a smile, she would not only please her guests, but also, unbelievably, herself.

Life is full of moments—make that hours—when we are beside ourselves with uncertainty, fear, stress, or any one of a host of dilemmas that weigh us down and paralyze our thoughts and actions. Sometimes we are under so thick a cloud of confusion that we are rendered immobile. Some people have found help through such means as prayer, meditation, or close friends. The innkeeper has her guests. What do you have?

How about the book you are holding in your hands? Like a guest knocking at your door, *365 Simple Pleasures* is bound to turn your day around.

By reading daily and trying out some of the suggestions, you will not only lift your spirits, but also experience pleasure and perhaps notice the same reaction as the innkeeper gets from her guests. You will come away feeling renewed and out of your sour mood. The point of Susannah Seton's new book on the exploration of comfort and joy in your life is that proactive, life-giving ideas are all around you, even in household chores. Sometimes, though, we are blind, as our minds race with so many things that we do not pay attention to what we are doing or how we are feeling.

Our author wants to bring us back to Earth, and she points out that past generations of women can help us get there. Pioneers were faced with making things by hand, and by doing so they were self-rejuvenated, an experience that we too can have. Bravo! Anything that brings us to our knees again will most assuredly also bring us to our senses, and thus to 365 pleasures and then some.

A BOWER OF PLEASURES

I 've been thinking and writing about simple pleasures for six years now, scouring old-fashioned crafts and recipe collections, hounding friends and family for ideas. What I've come to see is that in these mechanistic, commercial times, much joy can be found in reviving some of the traditions that our mothers, grandmothers, and great-grandmothers practiced in their homes in the name of necessity. Women in previous generations made their own bread, candles, and lotions because they had to; we in the twenty-first century have more choices about everything, and many of us are discovering that the choice to make a rosemary wreath rather than buy one or to make a batch of crackers from scratch is downright rejuvenating in some wonderfully fundamental way. Using our hands to make something—a homemade toss pillow, a jar of pickles—can be extremely pleasurable in and of itself—and that's not counting the pleasure to be derived from sharing it with others!

What you hold in your hands right now is 365 of these timeless pleasures—the little things that can make such a big difference in our lives and in the lives of those around us. They represent not only my ideas and stories, but those of hundreds of other folks as well. Not all these suggestions will appeal to you. Pleasure is extremely idiosyncratic; one person's delight might be another person's nightmare. But I hope you will find enough to bring you joy throughout the entire year.

Think of these offerings as a huge flower mart in which you get to wander, picking exactly the flowers you want to bring into your home to give you maximum delight. The idea is to enjoy yourself and to bring enjoyment to others, not to lay a guilt trip on yourself about how you should be more creative or take better care of yourself. In this, at least, if in no other corner of your life, it's all about savoring the simple beauty of being alive in the world.

—*Susannah Seton*

CREATE A SIMPLE PLEASURES LIST

What little things bring you joy? They're different for each of us. Here is my friend Pat's list: 1) when I really feel listened to; 2) when I have the bed all to myself; 3) when I take a hot bubble bath; 4) when my son gives me a big hug and holds on tight. Make your own list—and then be sure to indulge regularly.

BASIC WHITE BREAD

Nothing beats the smell of bread baking. It creates such a feeling of home!

1¼ cups low-fat milk, scalded
1½ tablespoons honey
1¼ teaspoons salt
2 tablespoons canola, corn, or safflower oil, plus a bit more

1¼ ounce package dry yeast
¼ cup warm water (105–115°)
3⅓ cups unbleached flour, approximately

Combine the first four ingredients in a large bowl. Stir and let cool to lukewarm. In a small bowl, dissolve yeast in warm water and add to milk mixture. Add flour to the mixture, a little at a time, to form a stiff dough. Mix well after each addition. Turn onto lightly floured board and kneed until smooth and elastic. Grease a large bowl and add dough, turning to grease top. Cover with damp towel. Let rise in a warm place until it has doubled in size. Punch down and let rest until it's doubled again. Punch down and let rest for 10 minutes. Shape into loaf and place in a greased 9-by-5-by-3-inch bread pan. Brush top with oil. Cover and let rise until it doubles in size. Preheat oven to 375°. Bake loaf until done, about 40 minutes. It should be brown on top and sound hollow when struck. Makes one loaf.

FRAYED-NERVES BATH

7 drops lavender essential oil
2 drops sweet marjoram essential oil
3 drops ylang-ylang essential oil

3

Fill tub with warm water, and then add oils. Swish the oils around in the water to evenly disperse them, then submerge yourself.

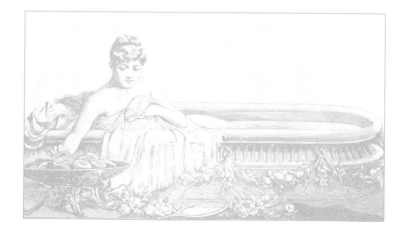

MAPLE CANDY

Heavy snowfalls are blessings for people who love maple candy. The good news is that you don't need an acre of sugar maples and a bucket of sap to make it: a bottle of maple syrup will do just fine.

½ cup maple syrup
1 baking pan full of packed, clean snow

Leave the pan of snow outside or in the fridge until you're ready to use it. Then heat the maple syrup in a pot to 270° (check with a candy thermometer). Carefully dribble the hot syrup in small patches over the snow. Each one of these patches will magically turn to maple candy. Yum!

PAINT WITH PASSION

Are you looking for an inexpensive way to jazz up your house? Add character to a room by painting the trim an unconventional color. If you are so inspired, consider the following: 1) Stay away from trendy colors—you're going to be living with them probably for a long time. And you might just want something different from what everyone else has. 2) Don't be afraid to mess up—you can always paint over it. 3) Think about the surrounding accent colors—will they mesh with the new color you've chosen?

CACTUS GARDEN

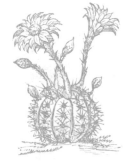

6

This makes a perfect gift for those who want plants but kill them by not watering them. Find a low ceramic pot or bowl and plant a few different varieties of cactus. You might want to add a pretty rock or dried flowers for color (red celosia is a wonderful choice). Handling a cactus doesn't have to be painful if you wrap a towel around it several times and use the towel like a noose to lift it out of the old pot and into the new. Rather than using your fingers, use a spoon to pack dirt around roots.

PERSONALIZED REFRIGERATOR MAGNETS

Can you ever have enough kitchen magnets? With all the stuff I tack up on my fridge, I certainly can't. Here's an easy way to make your own (and they're great gifts for Grandma that kids can make by themselves.) Save the metal lids from frozen drink cans. Find some favorite photos that will fit on the lids, and have color copies made of them. Cut the copies to fit, and using white glue or spray glue, affix the pictures to the lids, smoothing out any bubbles or wrinkles with your fingers. Glue a thin piece of ribbing around the edge and a magnet on the back. Presto!

CRANBERRY VINEGAR

You've heard of raspberry vinegar, but what about cranberry? It's great for using on salads and chicken dishes. Wash and pick over the cranberries and dry well on paper towels. Use 1 cup of fresh cranberries per quart of vinegar. Pack the cranberries into clean bottles or jars with lids or corks and fill with white wine vinegar that has been heated just to the boiling point. Cork or cap the bottles. Stand the jars on a sunny windowsill for about two weeks (four weeks if it's not very sunny). The warmth of the sun will infuse the vinegar with the cranberry flavor. Do a taste test; if the vinegar doesn't seem flavorful enough, strain it and add more cranberries. When it suits you, label and decorate the jars with a beautiful ribbon. Store at room temperature.

INDOOR GARDENS

In the winter when my garden is dry and bare, nothing gives me more pleasure than to visit the local garden shop, where it always feels like sweet, balmy summer. I wander through the rows of brightly colored flowers and richly hued shiny leaves, and the aroma of blossoms and sweet rich earth make me forget, for a time, the gloom and doom outside. The plants and flowers are completely oblivious to the weather outside, and their verdant outbursts of energy restore mine. I take an inordinate amount of time picking out some ridiculously expensive and riotously colored plant that just screams warm weather, which I take home and place on my windowsill or bedside table in a beautiful basket or brightly colored cachepot. I kind of have a "brown thumb," so my plants never last long, but I almost prefer that; it gives me a chance to go to the garden shop again that much sooner!

BRAENDENDE KAELIGHTED

This is Danish comfort food, designed to dispel the gloom of winter. Its name means "burning love." Fat phobics, beware!

1 pound potatoes, peeled and cut into chunks
8 to 10 slices bacon, chopped
3 onions, chopped
½ stick butter
½ pint cream (can substitute milk or low-fat milk)
salt, pepper, and nutmeg to taste

Cook the potatoes in water until tender. While the potatoes are cooking, fry the bacon with the onions until onions are tender. Drain potatoes and mash. Whip in butter and cream or milk. Season with spices. Mound potatoes on a plate and make a well in the center. Place bacon-onion mixture in the center. Serves 4.

VIRTUAL COOKING

If you are a great peruser of recipes, check out the site at www.kitchenlink.com. This site provides an exhaustive listing of recipes and food-related information. What I like about it is that you can type in a key word—let's say you have an abundance of broccoli and are looking for something different to do with it—and up pops a slew of recipes. Looking for low-fat or low-cal dishes? Check out www.fatfree.com and www.cyberdiet.com. If you are looking for a good place to buy natural food, don't miss Good Eats Shop-At-Home Natural Food at www.goodeats.com. And more than 6,000 recipes are available at www.epicurious.com, while wwwfoodchannel.com will link you to cooking contests, games, and restaurant reviews.

ROSEMARY WREATH

Rosemary grows in abundance in many parts of the country. I love to use it fresh, so I've learned to make this simple rosemary heart to hang in my kitchen. I just tear off sprigs as I need them. If I don't use it fast enough, no problem—it's just as tasty dried.

> 3 feet garden wire
> floral wire
> 12 long stems rosemary

Make a hook at heart end of the wire, then bend the wire into a heart shape and hook ends together. Starting at the top, attach a stem of rosemary to the wire with floral wire so that its leafy top points into the middle. Repeat on other side. Then wire stems down both sides and join at bottom. Makes 1 wreath.

SLEEP POTION

Here is a marvelous aromatherapy spray from Judith Fitzsimmons' and Paula M. Bousquet's wonderful book *Seasons of Aromatherapy*. Guaranteed to relax you and help you drift off.

2 drops chamomile essential oil
4 drops lavender essential oil
3 drops orange essential oil
5 ounces water

Mix all ingredients together in a spray bottle. Spray bed clothing and the air before bedtime.

THE NOSE KNOWS

What can compare to the smell of home cooking as you walk in the door after a hard day's work? I like it so much that I've taken to Crock-Pot cooking on my nights to cook so that the aromas will be awaiting me as soon as I hit the kitchen doorway. The new slow cookers are quite marvelous!

CHOCOLATE PUDDING

There is nothing like chocolate pudding made from scratch! It's actually quite simple to make. If you are a fan of the "skin" of the pudding, chill uncovered (the longer you chill it, the thicker it will get). If you dislike the skin, cover the pudding tightly and serve as soon as it's cold.

> 4 tablespoons cocoa
> 4 tablespoons cornstarch
> ⅔ cup sugar
> ¼ teaspoon salt
> 2 cups light cream
> 1 teaspoon vanilla extract

In the top of a double boiler over hot but not boiling water, combine cocoa, cornstarch, sugar, and salt. Add ½ cup cream and stir until smooth. Stir remaining cream in slowly, stirring constantly, until thick. Stir in vanilla. Pour into container and chill. Serves 4.

DON'T FORGET THE DIMMER

Why, when people are installing dimmers, do they always remember the bedroom, dining room, and living room but ignore the kitchen? Whenever I move, putting a dimmer in the kitchen is my first priority. That way, when guests come over and gather in the kitchen, as they invariably will, the lighting is as soft and flattering as it is in the rest of the house.

16

HOMEMADE BUBBLE BATH

Bubble bath is a great gift that even small kids can make. The trick is to have a pretty container to put it in and to never divulge your ingredients.

2 cups Ivory (or other unscented) dishwashing liquid
⅛ ounce of your favorite essential oil (vanilla is my favorite)

Drop the oil into the dishwashing liquid and let sit, covered for 1 week. Pour it into beautiful a bottle and add a gift tag and ribbon and instructions to use ¼ cup per bath. Enough for 8 baths.

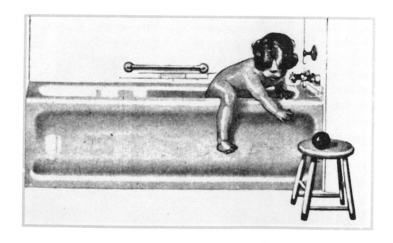

HANDMADE PRETZELS

Pretzels are great nonfat snacks that can easily be made at home. The longer you knead the dough, the softer the pretzel will be. If you've got kids, enlist them—to make the process more fun, the dough can easily be formed in the shapes of letters and numbers.

18

1½ cups warm water
1 package yeast
1 tablespoon sugar

4 cups flour
1 teaspoon salt, plus more for tops
1 egg, beaten

Preheat oven to 425°. Put the warm water into a large bowl, sprinkle in yeast, and stir until it dissolves. Add sugar, flour, and salt. Mix well, then knead dough until it is smooth and soft. Roll and twist dough into desired shapes—letters, numbers, twists, and so on. Grease two cookie sheets. Lay the pretzel dough shapes onto cookie sheets. Brush with beaten egg and sprinkle lightly with salt. Bake for 12 to 15 minutes, or until golden. Makes 1 to 2 dozen, depending on size.

THE LANGUAGE OF LOVE

Words do make the mood. We all know the usual terms of endearment—*honey, dear, sweetie, angel,* to name but a few. But to fan the flames of ardor and romance, why not try some less tired language, like *sweeting, sweetling,* or *sweetkin* (terms in vogue in the sixteenth and seventeenth centuries). Or how about *dearling* (the original form of *darling*)? Your partner could become your *paramour* (literally *through love*) in French. Instead of *attractive* or *cute,* you could try *toothsome* or *cuddlesome.* Rather than *missing,* try *yearning, pining, longing,* or *hungering,* and watch the passion build.

CRAZY FOR CRACKERS

Crackers are incredibly easy to make, and homemade ones are so much better than store-bought ones. I love sesame seeds, so I sprinkle some on just before baking—you can too!

> 2 cups all-purpose flour
> 1 teaspoon baking powder
> salt
> ¾ cup water, approximately
> sesame seeds, optional
> 4 tablespoons butter, margarine,
>   or other shortening

Preheat oven to 325°. Sift together flour, baking powder, and a pinch of salt. With 2 knives, cut the shortening into the flour until mixture is fine. Add just enough water to make a firm dough. On a lightly floured surface, roll out thinly with a floured rolling pin. Using a round cookie cutter, stamp out crackers, prick them all over with a fork, and sprinkle with salt and sesame seeds if desired. Bake on a lightly greased cookie sheet for 20 minutes or until crisp. Cool on a rack and store in airtight container. Makes 2 dozen.

SCENTED CANDLES

Surprise your sweetheart with a candlelit dinner for two with your own homemade scented candles gracing both the table and the bedroom. Their lovely fragrance will be released as they burn. Scented candles are incredibly easy to make—you just need to plan in advance. (If you haven't planned ahead, you can still get some of the effect by sprinkling a drop or two of your favorite essential oil in the melted wax of a plain candle as it burns.)

2 ounces of your favorite fragrance essential oil (or try a combination; vanilla and rose are my favorites for romance)
¼ cup orris root powder (available at herbal stores)
1 large airtight plastic container big enough to fit 6 candles
6 unscented candles, any size

Combine the oil(s) and the orris root and sprinkle in the bottom of the container. Place candles inside, cover, and store in a cool spot for 4 to 6 weeks.

TRACTOR TRACKS

After the first big blizzard of winter ends and the snow is clean and white, go outside and make tractor tracks. Walk with your feet pointing out at a 45-degree angle. First put your left foot down, then your right foot so that the heel is against the middle of your left foot, and then it's left, right, left till it looks just like a John Deere has passed through on the way to the barn. Don't forget to do both wheels, if you really want to impress your mom. To impress your kids, you may need to add a snow angel between the tracks. Just lie on your back and wave your arms back and forth in the snow. Get up carefully without stepping on your imprint. Admire your handiwork.

SNOW ICE CREAM

This is a wonderful nineteenth-century treat that you can replicate if you live in snowy climes.

1 cup heavy cream
¼ cup superfine sugar
2 teaspoons lemon extract
   or two tablespoons rosewater
8 to 10 cups fresh, clean snow

Mix the cream, sugar, and lemon extract or rosewater. Add the snow, beating with a whisk, using only enough snow to make a stiff ice cream. Serve immediately. Makes 8 servings.

OATMEAL MASKS

Masks are used to deep clean and condition the skin and should always be applied after you have thoroughly washed your face. Be sure to avoid your eyes. After applying, lie down for fifteen minutes, covering your eyes with water-moistened eye pads. The kind of mask you choose depends on your skin type. This one works for all types—and it's so easy to make.

½ cup water
¼ cup oatmeal

Bring water to a boil, add oats, and cook over medium heat about 5 minutes, stirring occasionally. Allow to cool until warm but not hot. Apply to clean skin and leave on for 15 minutes. Rinse with warm water, then cool.

BASKET OF LOVE

Do you want to surprise your paramour some evening? Make a love basket. Simply find a heart-shaped basket, spray-paint it red (sand it slightly first so the paint will stick better), add a pretty ribbon to the handle, and fill it with your beloved's favorite things: chocolate-covered cherries, sexy underwear—whatever he or she fancies. Then place it on your love's pillow to be discovered.

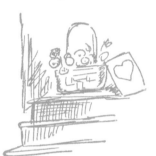

PERSONALIZED FURNITURE

26

You can create customized furniture that you and your kids will love. Find an old chest of drawers, a wooden trunk, or other wooden furniture at a garage sale. Paint it white or another solid color. Then dip baby's (older kids can do this themselves) hands and feet in water-based latex pastel paints and gently stamp them on the top and sides of the dresser. You'll have a permanent reminder of their childhood that you—and they—will treasure always.

THE PLEASURES
OF A GOOD BOOK

Read out loud to family members. When our kids are young, most of us do this naturally. But when children learn to read for themselves, we often give up this bonding activity. But we don't have to. No matter how old your child is, you can find something that you will both enjoy. Try it with your mate—I know a couple who read *Lord of the Rings* to each other and said that reading it together was much more fun than reading it on their own. Some people prefer reading and others being read to; find the combination that works for you.

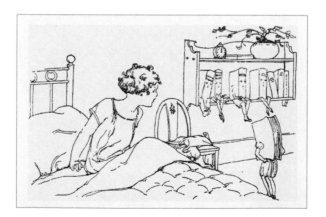

EYE PADS

These are great for those of us who use our eyes a lot—and who doesn't? Lie down for a quarter of an hour with these covering your eyes and presto—you'll feel rejuvenated in no time.

2 10-by-10-inch pieces of muslin
4 ounces dried chamomile flowers

With a pencil and ruler, mark off 2-inch squares on both pieces of fabric, with ⅜-inch seam allowances around each square. You should have 32 squares. Place one of the pieces of muslin down and put 1 teaspoon chamomile in the center of each square. Cover with the other piece of fabric and pin. Sew along the guidelines you have made for yourself. Cut apart. Makes 16. To use, place 2 in a small bowl and pour 1 table-spoon of boiling water over pads. Cover and let sit until luke-warm. Squeeze gently and apply to closed eyelids for 15 minutes.

CLEAN UP

In doing the *Simple Pleasures* series, I was struck by how many people wrote to tell me that some of their greatest pleasures were tidying, organizing, or cleaning some part of their homes. People mentioned straightening the tools in the garage, cleaning their desks before starting a new project, organizing the sock drawer once a year and throwing out all the single socks, and tackling the kitchen utensil drawer. What do you love to tidy or straighten up in your life? Give yourself a clean-up lift today.

FEAST OF WORDS

My idea of a good time these days is to stay in bed as long as possible in the morning reading a good book. Between working and parenting, I can never get enough of it. Sometimes I even wake up in the middle of the night and read for a couple hours just to get my fix. For my birthday, my husband entertained our daughter all day so that I could stay in bed with a thick thriller. What fun!

MEANINGFUL WALLPAPER

I read of a wonderful idea in *365 Days of Creative Play* by Sheila Ellison and Judith Gray. Just ask your child to draw pictures of the meaningful things in his or her life, like their hopes and dreams, beliefs, and loved ones. Then make a border at the top of your child's room with the pictures. It's a great way for a kid to decorate his or her own bedroom—and what a delight for you to look at.

31

HEARTFELT VALENTINE'S DAY

This year, rather than buying a card, why not make your loved ones personalized Valentine's Day cards? All you and/or your kids really need is imagination. To get started, consider the following:

- Look through a book of poetry to find just the right verse.
- Be brave and try expressing your thoughts directly.
- Take an 8½-by-11-inch piece of construction paper and fold in half. Keeping a ¼-inch margin at top and bottom of fold and between each design, cut little half-hearts and other designs in the fold. Open up and voilà! A homemade lace border.
- Decorate with lace doilies, glitter, dried flowers, and bits of ribbon.

LATE-NIGHT LOVE NOTES

Last Valentine's Day I started a new tradition with my husband. I gave him a little journal that was only to be used for writing love notes to each other. We keep it in the bedside table drawer, and whenever we feel compelled we make an entry then hide it under the other person's pillow. There's nothing like getting into bed, feeling that little lump under your head, and realizing that you have sweet words from your beloved to read before going to sleep.

33

SETTING THE SCENE

If you want great sex, think about creating a bedroom that's conducive to intimacy, says Will Ross in *The Wonderful Little Sex Book*. "It doesn't need to be elaborately furnished, but it should be uncluttered, have pleasing colors, and not be merely utilitarian; it should inspire a sense of beauty. The bed you use for sex ought to have a special, exotic, otherworldly feeling, almost evocative of an altar. There should be an air of reverence. Some people enjoy making love under a canopy, and you may want to construct one. Soft lighting is immensely helpful, and so is quietly pulsating music. When the whole room feels like a retreat from the hustle and bustle of everyday life, won't you relish the thought of spending time there with your beloved?"

GOOD BOOKS FOR
SENSUAL PLEASURE

In their book *Tantra: The Art of Conscious Loving,* teachers
Caroline and Charles Muir make the following suggestions
for a more meaningful connection: be love and nurture oriented, rather than goal oriented; be sure to give *and* receive,
and remember to make love a dance. Other good books on
sexual intimacy are *Soulful Sex* by Dr. Victoria Lee; *The Art
of Sexual Ecstasy* and *The Art of Sexual Magic* by Margo
Anand; and *Sexual Secrets* by Nik Douglas and Penny
Slinger.

HOPS FOR
A GREAT NIGHT'S SLEEP

Hops is said to be mildly sleep inducing, while lavender induces a sense of well-being. Together they make a great sleep pillow.

> 1 10-by-8-inch piece of muslin
> 4 handfuls dried hop flowers
> 2 handfuls dried lavender

Sew up three sides of the muslin and add the hops and lavender. Slip-stitch the open end. Pillow should be relatively flat. Makes 1 pillow.

CLEANING SOLUTIONS

Are you looking for assistance (the written kind) with cleaning every room in your house? Check out Jeff Campbell's *Household Solutions that Work* or www.thecleanteam.com on the Web. Consumer Reports' *How to Clean Practically Anything* is also great. If you want only nontoxic solutions, *Clean and Green* by Annie Berthold-Bond contains wonderful ideas that really work.

LAVENDER BATH POWDER

This is a delicious treat after a long soak in the tub.

⅛ cup dried lavender
mortar and pestle
1¼ cups cornstarch
25 drops lavender essential oil
small box and ribbon

With a mortar and pestle, grind the lavender into a fine dust. Mix together with the cornstarch. Stirring constantly, slowly add the essential oil drops and mix well. Place in a beautiful box and tie with a ribbon.

HOLD A COOKING PARTY

I love to gather a group of people to make something best done in an assembly line—cookies or tamales, for example. I buy all the ingredients, invite over neighbors or friends, open a bottle of wine, and cook, cook, cook. The time speeds by, the work goes quickly, and everyone goes home with a big pile of whatever we've made that afternoon. As far as I am concerned, a cooking party is the perfect blend of conviviality and cuisine.

39

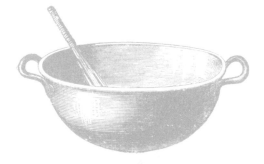

THE COMFY COUCH

What greater pleasure does life have to offer than a mid-afternoon Saturday nap on a comfy couch? Treat yourself to that delicious feeling you get when you know you should be up doing chores but instead are stretched out, luxuriating in doing absolutely nothing.

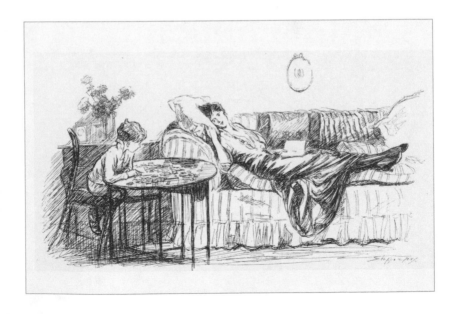

AROUND THE TABLE

I have a strict rule which I will break only for real emergencies—that my family sit down to dinner together at the dining room table every night. I mean, if we can't eat at least one meal a day together, why do we even call ourselves a family? It's our together time, the four of us around the table—telling jokes, sharing the news of our day. No TV, phone calls, video games, or books are allowed—just face-to-face interaction. One of the kids' favorite dinnertime conversations is what I call "remember when." Someone will start it: "Remember when I was two, Dad, and got the flu and threw up on you?" (The grosser the better for the kids.) "Remember when you where trying to hit the golf ball in the living room and broke Mum's best plant?" The half hour or so we spend together eating, talking, and laughing is what I remember most strongly when I look back over my life.

SKIN-SOOTHING BATH

Here's a great bath recipe for the winter, when skin gets so dry.

1 cup buttermilk
3 tablespoons Epsom salts
½ tablespoon canola oil
soothing essential oil of your choice,
    such as lavender or chamomile

Combine ingredients and pour into the stream of warm water as the tub is filling. Immerse yourself and relax for ten to fifteen minutes.

FLOWER FRAMES

You can beautify family photos by matting them with attractive colored mats and then gluing on dried flowers. A great gift!

Mat frames
Spanish moss
dried flowers
glue gun

Find mats that fit the photos you want to frame. Arrange the moss and flowers in an attractive pattern on the mat, and then hot-glue in place.

THE DELIGHTS OF SCENT

From time immemorial, scent has been used as an aphrodisiac. Time-tested fragrances include amber, ambergris, jasmine, lily of the valley, musk, myrrh, orange blossom, patchouli, sandalwood, and tuberose. Contemporary "erotically oriented" perfumes include Eau Sauvage, Magic Noire, and Poison, each of which contain some of these ancient aphrodisiacs. You might also try using essential oils in a diffuser in the bedroom or burning incense.

HEART PLACEMATS

These lovely placemats will grace your table for months to come.

tracing paper
Scotch tape
2 15-by-19-inch pieces of washable fabric, red or
  patterned with hearts
thread to match
straight pins

Tape 2 8½-by-1-inch pieces of tracing paper together along the 8½-inch sides. Fold in half along the tape seam and cut out a heart. Open and trace this heart on the wrong side of the fabric pieces. Cut out. Place the two sides of the heart together, right side in. Pin. Stitch along the outside of the heart, ¼ inch from edge, leaving an opening of about two inches. Clip along curved edges and in crevice. Turn right side out and slip stitch the opening. Makes 1 placemat.

HAIR MOISTURIZER

Rosemary is very good for hair, particularly dark hair, to which it imparts a wonderful shine. It will also help cut down on the problem of flyaway hair. This recipe makes enough for several applications.

8 drops cedar essential oil
8 drops lavender essential oil
12 drops rosemary essential oil
2 tablespoons olive oil

In a small glass container, mix the essential oils together. Add the olive oil. Pour about a teaspoon into the palm of your hand and rub hands together. Massage your head, hair, and scalp with the blend. Put a shower cap or warm towel on your head and leave it on for fifteen minutes. Wash and rinse your hair twice.

GARLIC SPREAD

Years ago independent filmmaker Les Blank made a movie called *Garlic Is as Good as Ten Mothers*. If you agree, you should try this confit. Slather it on sourdough baguettes or use it any time a recipe calls for cooked garlic. And don't forget to use the leftover garlic-infused oil. If you have a large garlic crop or make a trip to the farmers' market, you can package this up in gift jars for friends as well as for yourself.

> 8 ounces garlic cloves, peeled
> 2 cups olive oil
> sterilized jars with lids that seal

In a medium saucepan, bring the garlic and oil to simmer and cook over low heat for 25 to 30 minutes or until garlic is very tender. Cool and pack into containers. Store in refrigerator and use within two weeks. Makes 2 pounds.

PINE BATH OIL

This oil is a great skin softener. Just pour a bit into your bath under the running water.

1 cluster pine needles
1 cup baby oil, approximately

Put the pine needles in a glass container with a lid. Cover completely with baby oil and cover tightly. Store in dry, cool place for 4 weeks. Strain the oil, and decant into attractive glass bottle. If you'd like, you can add fresh pine needles for decoration. Makes 1 cup.

MAD FOR MUSHROOMS?

Gardeners who need a fix during the cold winter months should consider a mushroom kit. These kits come in a number of varieties, including shiitake and button. The kits contain a sterilized, enriched growing medium that is preinoculated with mushroom spawn that can easily be grown indoors in a cool, dark place year round. Shiitake, oyster, and portobello mushroom kits are available from Real Goods (800-762-7325), Gardener's Supply Company (800-863-1700), and Edmund Scientific Co. (609-573-6250). Edmund offers a catalogue with more than 4,000 science products, including lots of other kits. Great for science-minded kids.

I COULD HAVE
DANCED ALL NIGHT

This is something I do only when I'm alone. I put old Bob Marley tapes on my stereo and dance by myself in the living room. Sometimes I watch myself in the mirror. But mostly I dance with my eyes closed, just feeling the music as it moves through my body. Of course, you need to pick the music and the circumstances that are just right for you. Give it a try and see how it makes you feel.

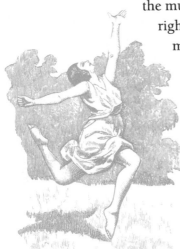

MEXICAN HOT CHOCOLATE

This drink is fabulous, the perfect thing for a cold evening.
If you have cinnamon-flavored Ibarra chocolate, use it instead of the semisweet and omit the cinnamon and brown
sugar.

51

4 cups milk
3 3-inch long cinnamon sticks, broken in half
30 whole cloves
1 teaspoon aniseed
5 ounces semisweet chocolate, chopped
2 tablespoons unsweetened cocoa powder
2 tablespoons brown sugar

In a large, heavy saucepan over medium heat, bring the milk,
cinnamon, cloves, and aniseed to a simmer. Add the remaining
ingredients and whisk until the chocolate melts. Remove from
heat, cover, and let steep for 45 minutes. Serves 4.

CALMING BATH

The sensual delight of taking a bath in aromatic oils goes back to the Romans, who raised bathing to a high art. The public baths consisted of three parts: first you went to the unctuarium, where you were anointed in oils. Then you proceeded to the frigidarium, where you took a cold bath, then to the tepidarium for a tepid one. You finished with a hot bath in the caldarium. While we don't bathe as the Romans did, we can indulge in the essence of the practice.

4 drops bergamot essential oil
4 drops lavender essential oil
2 drops clary sage essential oil

Run a warm bath. Drop the essential oils into the stream of water. Slide in, and relax for 10 to 15 minutes.

CANDY-COATED FUN

I keep a great big candy bowl on my desk at work. Most of my co-workers eventually end up there at some point in the day, rummaging through the bowl for their favorites. I always keep it filled with a variety of small, individually wrapped items—bubble gum, fireballs, peppermints, lifesavers, chocolate, and lollipops—and make sure it's all fresh. They enjoy the candy, and I enjoy the visits!

53

LOVE CLOTH

For her son's first birthday, a friend of mine bought a white linen tablecloth. She has since used it only on his birthday. She invites guests at each year's birthday party to sign their names (or, in the case of toddlers, to draw something, which she then signs) on his tablecloth with permanent markers. Now, ten years later, she has a colorful tablecloth full of memories that will last a lifetime. The kids love writing on it and reading all the messages from past birthdays.

GO WILD—AT LEAST A LITTLE

Sometimes we just need to shake up our routine. What little outrageous thing can you do today? Dye your hair? Paint your toenails green? Play hooky from work? For years, I lived near a street that must have had six or seven Chinese restaurants, and over time, I've probably eaten at them all. One day, I commented to my husband that each seemed to do a particular dish well and that putting them all together would make a great meal. So one night, when we were feeling the need to be a bit outrageous, we did just that. We had potstickers from one place, then moved onto the next for hot and sour soup, a third for the Szechwan beef, and a fourth for the garlic eggplant. If anyone thought we were weird only ordering one item per restaurant, no one said anything. We had a ball—not to mention a great dinner.

CANDLE COLLARS

A wonderful way to dress up pillar candles is to make a candle collar. The candle must be fat enough to be safe, and you should never leave it unattended. Make sure you place the candle on a dish so that the hot wax won't spread all over and snuff out the candle, with an inch left at the bottom of the collar to avoid accidents.

> bay leaves, magnolia leaves,
>   or other attractive oval-shaped leaves
> glue gun
> pillar candle
> raffia

Put a little glue on the back of each leaf near the base and press firmly to the candle. Trim the bottom of the leaves so that the candle stands evenly. Tie raffia around in a bow. Makes 1 candle.

FACIAL SAUNA

2 drops fennel essential oil
2 drops lavender essential oil
2 drops lemon essential oil
2 drops orange essential oil

Mix oils together and pour into a bowl of steaming water. Drape a towel over your head and the bowl and sit, allowing the steam to penetrate your pores. Be careful not to put your face too close—this should be luxurious, not a painful experience!

CRANBERRY TEA

This is a wonderfully spicy potion. The recipe makes enough for a crowd. You can make it with decaf bags if you want to avoid the kick.

4 cups water
4 cups cranberry juice
4 orange pekoe tea bags
¾ teaspoon cinnamon
16 cloves
1 apple, cored, seeded, and cut into 8 slices

Bring water and juice to a boil over medium heat. Place the tea bags in the mixture, cover, and remove from heat. Let steep 10 minutes. Remove the bags. Add the cinnamon. Place 2 cloves in each apple slice and add to tea. Let steep 5 minutes. Pour into mugs, making sure each cup gets 1 apple slice. Serves 8.

HOMEMADE FIRE STARTERS

Here's a great gift for anyone with a fireplace or woodstove.

> 1 block paraffin
> food dye
> pine or cedar essential oil
> several medium or large pinecones
> old tongs
> waxed paper

59

Melt the paraffin in the top of a double boiler. Add dye of your choice to color the wax and a few drops of pine or cedar essential oil to scent. Stir with an old wooden spoon. Using tongs, dip pinecones in wax to cover, and then set on waxed paper to harden.

ALL-PURPOSE ROOM SPRAY

When the house feels musty and stale, try this aromatherapy spray to freshen things up a bit. The authors of *Seasons of Aromatherapy* also recommend adding a few drops to your laundry to freshen up the clean clothes.

4 drops lavender essential oil
2 drops peppermint essential oil
2 drops tea tree essential oil
2 cups water

Combine all ingredients in a spray bottle. Spray your rooms.

COAXING SPRING

When you've got the winter blahs, one of the easiest cures is to anticipate spring by forcing branches to bring a bit of color indoors. Any of a wide variety of bushes, shrubs, and trees will do, including forsythia, crab apple, pussy willows, quince, cherry, plum, pear, dogwood, privet, red maple, gooseberry, weeping willow, and witch hazel. Simply cut the edges of the branches on a slant with sharp scissors and plunge immediately into a vase of warm water. As the days pass, make sure to keep the vases filled with plenty of clean, tepid, and the warmth of the house will do the rest of the work. Voilà—instant spring!

MAKE A PLAY DATE

My friend Daphne and I love to play dress up. We go shopping just for fun and often don't buy a thing. We just spend a few hours trying on clothes and seeing how we look in them. Ballgowns are particularly enjoyable; just the other day we found the perfect thing for Daphne to wear to the Academy Awards if she were ever invited. She looked just like Marilyn Monroe at J. F. K.'s birthday party. How do you like to play? Do you like mountain biking? Wind surfing? Going to a spa and having a facial? Do something you think of as play today.

EXOTIC POTPOURRI

If you're in the mood to give your living room an exotic scent, using the following potpourri is a wonderful way to do just that. This recipe makes a lot, but it is very long lasting and makes a great gift.

1 cup orris root
2 teaspoons rose oil
4 cups dried rose petals
4 cups vetiver root or vetivert
3 cups patchouli leaves
1 cup sandalwood
2 cups mace

Using a wooden spoon, combine the orris root and rose oil in a large nonmetallic bowl. Add the remaining ingredients and pack into boxes or jars. Let set for 4 weeks, shaking occasionally. Makes 14 cups.

FAMILY HOME EVENING

At one point I grew tired of running all over with all the kids every day—to soccer practice, games, piano lessons, tennis, play dates with friends. . . the list went on and on. I was exhausted, and the kids seemed cranky; there was never any downtime. It seemed as if we never had an evening to spend together as a family. Then I read about the tradition that Mormons have of a weekly "family home evening" and decided that was just what our family needed. And so I decreed Wednesdays as our home evening. After dinner, all of us spend the evening together with the TV off and with no outsiders, meetings, classes, or other commitments. Sometimes we play cards or a board game, read a story aloud, or tell ghost stories; other times we bake cookies together or just read in the same room. The kids protested at first, but now they too have gotten into the spirit.

THE PARTY FAN

Creatively folded napkins add to the beauty of any place setting. Here's a folding method that takes no time at all. If you don't have napkin rings, use a bit of ribbon or raffia as a tie. First, fold the napkin in half to form a horizontal rectangle. Fold the rectangle into 1-inch accordion pleats, and put on the ring or ribbon. Then spread out the pleats at the top and bottom to create a fan.

HOMEMADE STICKERS

If you have kids under the age of twelve, chances are they love stickers. And stickers can be mighty expensive. But you can make your own by turning any picture you want into a sticker. Collect appropriate images. Then, in a small cup, mix 2 parts white glue and 1 part vinegar. Use a small paintbrush to brush the mixture on the back of the picture. Let dry 1 hour, then cut, lick, and stick. The advantage to homemade stickers is that kids will have a ball making them!

CANDLE-MAKING SUPPLIES

Most hobby and craft stores carry everything you need to make candles of all sorts. But if you have trouble finding what you need, contact Barker Enterprises in Seattle at (206-244-1870). They have all kinds of supplies, including more than 650 candle molds. Other good sources are CandlechemCo. in Massachusetts (617-986-7541); Pourette Manufacturing in Seattle (800-800-WICK); and Charlotte Hobbys in Quebec (516-247-2590).

67

GOOD FOR WHAT AILS YOU

If you suffer from menstrual cramps or premenstrual discomfort, you may find the following bath remedy to be soothing and calming. The water will dilate your blood vessels and relax your muscles, while the herbs provide aromatherapy.

> 2 tablespoons dried lavender
> 2 tablespoons dried rose petals
> 3 tablespoons dried chamomile
> 2 tablespoons hops

Combine the herbs in a glass or ceramic bowl and pour in a quart of boiling water. Cover and let sit for an hour. Strain the herbs and pour under the running tap of a warm (not hot) bath.

FREE VACATION

When my husband is away, I sometimes spend the night in the guest bedroom in the old-fashioned double bed I used before I was married. It has a fluffy comforter, ruffled pillow shams, and pretty sheets. If I adjust the miniblinds just right, I get a lovely view of the treetops and city lights, a nice contrast to the tar-and-gravel rooftops and power lines I see during the day. And because there is only one outlet in the room, just enough for a lamp and a clock, I read in bed instead of watching TV. Spending the night in the guest room makes me feel as though I'm staying at a bed and breakfast. As Jane Austen once said, "There is nothing like staying at home for real comfort."

69

HERBAL SOAP BALLS

Here's an easy, inexpensive homemade gift that the little ones can help with. The kids will love the pulverizing, and recipients will like its clean fragrance.

> 1 tablespoon dried herbs, pulverized (you can use rosemary, sage, thyme, peppermint, or a combination)
> 5 drops matching essential oil
> 1 personal-size Ivory soap bar, shredded and placed in a mixing bowl

Pour ¼ cup boiling water over the herbs and add the essential oil. Let steep for 20 minutes. Bring this mixture to a boil and pour over the soap. When cool enough, mix well by hand and let stand for 15 minutes. Mix again and form into 3 balls. Place on plastic wrap and let stand for 3 days. Makes 3 soap balls.

HOMEMADE FLOUR TORTILLAS

My husband swears by these.

> 4 cups flour
> 1¼ teaspoon salt
> 6 tablespoons vegetable shortening
> approximately 1¼ cups boiling water

Sift together the flour and salt into a large bowl. Mix the shortening in by hand until the mixture resembles cornmeal and feels slightly gritty to the touch. Stir in enough boiling water that the dough sticks together. Place the dough on a floured surface and knead for approximately 5 minutes. Form dough into a ball, place inside the bowl, and cover with plastic wrap. After approximately 30 minutes, divide the dough into 10 to 12 balls, and roll each flat with a well-floured rolling pin. Cook in a cast-iron skillet over medium heat, about 20 seconds on each side. Makes 10 to 12 tortillas.

THE PLEASURE
OF GIVING PLEASURE

Pleasing someone else is a pleasure like no other. Cook a special dish for your mate, find the perfect sweater for a friend, treat your child to her favorite ice cream. Today, indulge someone else in his or her simple pleasure and notice how good it makes you feel.

SCENTED NOTEPAPER

We all send letters so infrequently these days that when we do, it should be a pleasurable experience for both the sender and the receiver. You can add a romantic touch to your personal correspondence by scenting your stationery. It's incredibly easy. This recipe makes enough for you and your friends.

>   8 ounces unscented talcum powder
>   15 drops of your favorite essential oil or perfume
>   6 small, closely woven cotton or silk bags, open on one side
>   ribbon
>   notepaper and envelopes
>   1 plastic bag

In a bowl, combine the powder and perfume. Cover tightly and let sit for a day. Spoon the mixture into the bags and tie with ribbon. Place the bags in between the layers of notepaper and envelopes in a box and put the box into the plastic bag. Allow to sit for a few days so that the scent will permeate the paper. Makes 6 sachets.

INDOOR GREENERY

When it's gray and dreary outside, I like to plant an indoor kitchen garden in a sunny window. One of my favorites is a lemon herb garden, because it lends such a tart fragrance to the room. You can either put plants in one long container or use a variety of small pots. Choose from lemon basil, lemon verbena, lemon thyme, lemon balm, lemon geranium, and lemongrass to fill the air with the delicious, tangy scent of citrus. Treat these plants to plenty of sun and well-drained soil. Be sure to pick the blooms off of lemon verbena and lemon basil. The more you pick and use these herbs, the more prolific the plants will be. Consider mixing in a yellow flowering plant to visually highlight the lemon fragrance. What to do with all this lemon flavor? Try making lemon honey: Coarsely chop ½ cup lemon balm or lemon verbena and place in a saucepan with 1 cup honey. Over low heat, cook for 20 minutes, then strain out herbs and store honey in a container with a tight lid. Or make lemon butter: Soften ½ cup butter and mix in 2 tablespoons of finely chopped lemon basil or lemon thyme. Great for seafood and pasta.

AN EASY PICK-ME-UP

When the winter doldrums really grip your family, how about hosting a slumber party for all your children's friends? They will love it, and even if it gives you a sleepless night, at least you won't be bored. To make it a night to remember, buy inexpensive plain pillowcases and have the kids sign them with permanent markers. Provide a variety of colors for artistic inspiration. Parents can later stitch over the names if they want and have a keepsake.

FLOWER BARRETTES

These are wonderful for kids of all ages.

> plain plastic hair barrettes
> small dried flowers—
>   (small rose buds and baby's breath are nice)
> glue gun

Decide on a pleasing arrangement, and hot-glue the flowers onto the barrettes.

GOING OUT FOR BREAKFAST

My father was an old-fashioned country doctor who made house calls and visited his patients in the county hospital every day except Sunday. On Saturdays, he would get up early and, on the way to the hospital, stop for breakfast at what my mother always referred to as "the dirty diner." It was a greasy spoon in an old railroad car with split black leather booths whose chief appeal to my dad was the break in his routine of coffee and the newspaper before rushing off to work. I too have learned the pleasure of a regular breakfast out. It's a chance to slow down and observe the start of the day through new eyes. Also, eating a good breakfast is good for you both mentally and physically. So go to a café and sit among people you normally don't see. You can still read the newspaper, but remember to listen to new sounds and conversation and enjoy the smells that only breakfast provides.

SENSUAL BATH

This bath feels luxurious beyond belief.

2 drops cedar essential oil
2 drops clary sage essential oil
2 drops lavender essential oil
2 drops orange essential oil
2 tablespoons vegetable oil

Combine all oils and pour the mixture into the stream of a warm bath.

INSTANT GOURMET

You can easily make your own flavored olive oils. Buy some decorative bottles or use recycled wine bottles. Be sure to use only fresh herbs, to wash them well, to make sure the oil completely covers all the ingredients, and to seal the bottle tightly and use within three weeks. Because garlic contains the spores for a bacteria that, when added to oil, can cause botulism, it's best not to make any garlic-flavored oil (the store-bought kind uses sterilized garlic.) To make chili oil, simply add 5 yellow Thai chilies and 1 teaspoon peppercorns to 5 cups of olive oil, cap the bottle tightly, and let stand in a cool place for a week. For lemon pepper oil, slice a lemon for each bottle you plan to make and dry in oven at 170° for about 5 hours, or until dry but not crisp. To a bottle of oil, add 1 tablespoon whole black peppercorns and the slices from one dried lemon. For rosemary oil, add 3 large sprigs of rosemary to a bottle of olive oil.

INDULGE IN DINNER

It's easy to get the winter blues. I remember when I lived in Ithaca, New York, it could be overcast for six weeks or more at a time during the winter. By March I was really down. So to combat the winter blues, take the opportunity tonight to indulge yourself with a really good dinner. Make your favorite food. Buy fresh flowers, use cloth napkins, light a scented candle. Go all out for no other reason than to enjoy yourself.

EASY HERBAL BOUQUET

When purchasing fresh herbs, cut off the bottoms and place them in a nice vase on the kitchen sill. This not only brightens up the kitchen, but it also adds fragrance, keeps the herbs fresher longer, and has the added benefit of reminding you to use them in a variety of dishes.

BUTTERFLY KISSES

Give someone you love butterfly kisses on the cheek today. (And maybe you'll get some in return. Either way is luscious.) In case you don't know how to do it, it's easy—simply flutter your eyelashes across your intended's cheek.

ART PILLOW

You can't needlepoint, quilt, sew, or crochet? Don't worry. making a one-of-a-kind pillow for your living room is as easy as pie—all you need is a drawing that you or your child has done and a few items from a fabric store.

1 drawing
1 pillow-sized piece of foam
2 pieces of plain fabric, each an inch larger
   around than the foam
tracing paper
liquid embroidery (available at craft stores)
needle and thread

Trace the drawing onto one of the pieces of fabric. Using the liquid embroidery, embroider the lines of the drawing onto the fabric. Place the two pieces of fabric together inside out and sew on three sides. Insert the foam and stitch the fourth side.

PERSONALIZED WRAPPING PAPER

You and your family can make your own wrapping paper. Buy a roll of white butcher paper or brown paper. For ease, you can purchase a few rubber stamps and different colored ink pads, and simply stamp out a pattern on your paper. Be careful not to smear the ink as you go. To make the paper even more personalized, you can make your own rubber stamps. Cut a potato in half, carve a simple shape into the center, then cut the sides away so your center design is elevated enough to make a clear impression. Try simple shapes like hearts, stars, dots, and diamonds. For simple polka dots you can use wine corks. What's great is that everyone gets to express his or her individuality.

HEAVENLY HAM

This is a classic recipe that has graced many Easter, Thanksgiving, and Christmas tables. If you have managed to live this long without giving it a try, rectify the situation immediately (if you eat ham!). You're guaranteed to be delighted.

> 1 ham, about 5 pounds
> whole cloves
> brown sugar
> 1 20-ounce can pineapple slices in juice
> maraschino cherries

Preheat oven to 350°. Score the surface of ham with a knife and insert whole cloves in each intersection. Put in baking pan and bake. If ham is not precooked, allow 20 minutes per pound. If precooked, follow wrapper instructions. Pour juice from pineapple slices into a bowl. Add enough brown sugar to make a thin paste. Baste ham with glaze every 15 minutes or so. Cover the ham with the pineapple rings approximately half an hour before ham is done (use toothpicks to hold in place if necessary), and place a cherry in the center of each pineapple slice. Serves 8.

DECORATIVE CHOKER

Dressing up in all your finery is fun, especially when the weather turns warm. This easy-to-make necklace is perfect for young girls and women of all ages.

velvet ribbon
1-inch length of self-stick Velcro
  (should be the same color as the ribbon)
scissors
dried flower
spray craft glaze
hot glue

Measure the neck size of the wearer. Add 1 inch and cut the ribbon to this size. Take the fuzzy-cloth side of the Velcro and attach it to one end of the ribbon (if the backing is not strong enough to attach to the ribbon, use a drop of hot glue). Take the plastic side of the Velcro and cut it in half. Attach this to the backside of the other end of the ribbon. Make sure that when you wrap the ribbon around the person's neck the Velcro catches. Take the dried flower and spray the head with the glaze to protect it. After it has dried, cut off the stem. Hot-glue the flower to the center of the ribbon.

RESTORE A PIECE OF FURNITURE

Because so many of us work primarily with our heads, doing something with our hands can be tremendously satisfying. I have an old pine blanket chest that I bought about twenty years ago. Over the years it has endured dog scratches, children's scribbles, and scrapes from candleholders. One day I decided it needed some help. So I sanded it down a bit and applied coat after coat of Briwax and then cream furniture polish. Now it glows again, and I smile every time I walk into the room. Find something with intrinsic quality and value. If someone once cared about the piece, no matter how many layers of paint and neglect it has endured, you can restore it. Enjoy your creativity and a sense of preserving the past. Or do what my co-worker Brenda does. Find a junky wooden or metal chair that is being thrown away and save it from the landfill. Use your imagination and paint it to have a one-of-a-kind creation. Each leg a different color? The sky on the seat? Let your imagination soar.

INDULGE IN A HEAD MASSAGE

Giving a head massage is easy and requires no formal training. All you need is someone who enjoys getting his or her head rubbed and is willing to reciprocate. Stand behind the person and place your hands very gently on his head. Just rest there for a few seconds; the idea is for the two of you to relax together and for you to get in tune with him. If it is comfortable for him, have him close his eyes. Place both hands on top of his head, so they meet at the midline. Using all your fingers, press and massage in circular motions, covering the entire scalp from forehead to nape of neck, and from ear to ear. Ask him to guide you as to how much pressure to apply. Use your thumbs on the spot where the base of the skull meets the neck. Massage his temples in a firm, circular motion for a minute. Slowly massage your way across the forehead until your hands meet in the middle. Return to the temples and bring your hands down either side of her head to the point in front of the earlobes where the jaw tends to clench. Massage there. Finish off by gently pulling on his hair and tugging upward.

INDULGE YOUR
INNOCENT CRAVING

I have a confession: I love Coca-Cola, as in six-cans-a-day-if-I-didn't-control-myself. For many years after my college Coke bingeing, I resisted altogether. Then I married someone with the same secret passion, and it crept back into the house. I wavered, worried, and finally decided that I could enjoy one Coke a day at most, no more. And I've kept to my commitment for years. Many days I have none, but when I do choose to have one, I really enjoy it. I drink it consciously, noticing the bubbles as it goes down my throat, the cold sweetness on my tongue. I savor my Coke, wringing every drop of pleasure out of it.

Just for today, indulge your innocent craving (this is not permission for alcoholics to drink, food addicts to eat, or ex-potheads to smoke; I'm talking harmless non-addictive pleasures)—the Chunky Monkey ice cream; the chocolate cake with mocha frosting; the bananas with peanut butter. Whatever it is that you love to eat but avoid because you are being good, go ahead and splurge. And while you're splurging, really relish it.

OLD-FASHIONED RICE PUDDING

Here's a warming treat, especially good for the March doldrums. And it couldn't be easier to make.

3½ cups milk
½ cup sugar, divided into 2¼ cups
½ teaspoon cinnamon
½ cup long-grain rice
2 egg yolks
½ cup whipping cream
1 teaspoon vanilla

Heat milk, ¼ cup sugar, and cinnamon in saucepan just to boil; stir in rice and reduce heat to low. Cover and simmer for 35 to 45 minutes. In a separate bowl, whisk egg yolks, cream, ¼ cup sugar, and vanilla. Add gradually to rice. Bring to a boil and cook, stirring, for 3 minutes longer. Makes 4 servings.

LACY BEAUTY

Make lace napkin rings for your cloth napkins. Simply roll the napkins and tie with 24 inches of 1-inch-wide lace. Trim edges of the lace so they look finished.

GET INTO HOT WATER

Remember Fizzies? You'd drop tablets in a glass of water, and they would turn into a bubbly fruit drink. Well, now someone has invented some for the bathtub. Drop one in your tub and watch the fizzy bubbles rise. The secret ingredient? Baking soda, which happens to be good for your skin as well as fun in the tub. Brand names include Bath Fizzies, Bath Bombs, Get Fresh!, and Bath Bloomers Botanical Pollens.

CITRUS TONER

This toner is great for oily or normal skin.

¼ cup lemon peel, finely grated
¼ cup grapefruit peel, finely grated
1 cup mint leaves
1 cup water

Add mint and citrus peelings to rapidly boiling water. Continue to boil for 1 to 2 minutes or until peels become soft and slightly translucent. Remove from heat. Cool and strain. Store in the refrigerator or freezer; it will last 2 to 3 weeks.

USE GOOD SCENTS

Smells can be mood elevators. Here are some ways to bring good scents into your day. Light a candle with a favorite scent before you go to bed, letting it perfume the room. My favorite is Casablanca lily. Jasmine is a good choice too; it induces optimism. Just be sure to blow out the candle before you fall asleep. Apply a scented lotion or one or two drops of your favorite essential oil to your temples and rub gently. Various body stores even have specialized "pulse point" lotions.

FLOATING CANDLES

Candles add a magical element to any room. I especially love using the floating ones as a centerpiece for the dining room table, solving the problem of having an arrangement that interferes with conversation. Simple float a few candles and some flowers in a bowl, and you have an elegant focal point.

12 ounces paraffin
60 drops your favorite essential oil
12 1-inch floating candlewicks
(available at craft stores)
12 metal pastry tins or candle molds

In a double boiler, melt the paraffin and then add the essential oil with a wooden spoon. Pour wax into molds slowly to avoid air bubbles. Let half set and then insert wicks in the center of each. Let candles set fully and then unmold. Makes 1 dozen.

FOR THE LOVE OF BOOKS

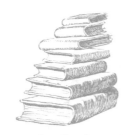 If your head feels full of fog and you haven't had an interesting conversation with anyone recently, consider joining or starting a book club. Many bookstores run several groups (and may even offer discounts if you all buy your books through the store), and community newsletters often run classifieds with groups looking for new members. Most groups we know are made up of friends who use the club as a way to get together regularly. You need enough people to make your group interesting and to accommodate the vagaries of people's schedules. Six to eight is a good ballpark figure. Usually groups rotate who picks the book for the next meeting; some groups have length limits. Many book group guides exist to help you pick books, provide discussion topics, and offer suggestions. Check with your local bookstore.

CANDLE POTS

One of the easiest and most attractive arrangements you can make for a table or sideboard is a series of cream or white pillar candles in terra-cotta pots. Just group them attractively, and you have a simple yet sophisticated feeling. Make sure you never leave candles unattended; the moss can catch on fire if the candle burns too far down.

> Dry floral foam
> 1 terra-cotta pot
> 1 pillar candle
> glue gun
> green, sphagnum, or reindeer moss
> floral or straight pins

Trim the foam to approximately the same shape as the pot, making sure it is a little larger than the pot's diameter. Push the foam firmly into the pot until it touches the bottom. Trim if needed to get a good fit. Pack the spaces around the foam with moss. Trim top of foam level with pot. Glue candle to foam. Surround base of candle with moss, fixing it in place with pins. Makes 1.

TIME CAPSULE

A family I know recently made a family time capsule and all three kids—ages five, seven, and twelve—really enjoyed it. They took an old trunk, and each person put in something to represent themselves, something they considered important. They put in the day's newspaper, a grocery store receipt (the twelve-year-old's idea to compare prices now and then), and photos of themselves they had recently taken. Then they sealed it and put a note on top saying they would open it in 2015. They all had a great time together deciding what to include.

MINTCENSE

Originally made in colonial times, when it was believed to "clear the head," mint potpourri makes an excellent natural room freshener. The following was taken from a recipe by Phyllis Shaudys, who says the concoction sells well at craft fairs.

½ cup orris root
½ tablespoon oil of
  lavender or pennyroyal
2 cups dried orange mint
2 cups dried spearmint
2 cups dried peppermint
1 cup dried thyme
1 cup dried rosemary

Combine the orris root and essential oil. Add the rest of the ingredients and combine gently, taking care not to crush the leaves too much. Store in a covered jar. To use, shake and open.

APRIL SHOWERS

My favorite household chore is giving my indoor plants their yearly spring shower. I carry them all outside and thoroughly hose them off with water, sometimes hand washing individual leaves if they are particularly dusty. Then I pluck dead leaves and bulbs, trim brown ends with scissors, and replace old soil with fresh if needed. When I return the plants indoors, they sparkle so much I could swear they were thanking me.

BUTTERFLY HAVEN

If you want to increase the butterfly population in your yard this summer, you can plant a wide variety of flowers to attract them, including common yarrow, New York aster, Shasta daisy, coreopsis, horsemint, lavender, rosemary, thyme, butterfly bush, shrubby cinquefoil, common garden petunia, verbena, pincushion flowers, cosmos, zinnia, globe amaranth, purple coneflower, sunflowers, lupine, and delphinium. Keep in mind that butterflies also need wind protection, a quiet place to lay eggs, and drinking water.

If you want to see a butterfly garden before you get started, many botanical societies have them. In Washington, D.C., the Smithsonian just opened one adjacent to the National Museum of Natural History. Good guides include *The Butterfly Garden* by Matthew Tekulsky (Harvard Common Press) or *Butterfly Gardening* by Xerces Society/Smithsonian Institution (Sierra Club Books).

DO SOMETHING YOU LOVE

What gives you great pleasure that you haven't done in a while? Going to the movies and eating a large bucket of popcorn? Reading a trashy novel? Calling a friend long distance? Whatever it is, give yourself permission to indulge today.

EGGSHELL PLANTERS

Ordinary eggshells make beautiful planters for small herbs or grasses. Break raw eggs, leaving shell at least one half intact. Empty the contents into a separate bowl, and rinse the shell thoroughly. Place already sprouting plants (mint, lavender, chives, or sage work well, as does wheat grass, alfalfa, or small ferns) in the shells, anchored with a bit of topsoil. Cushion an assortment of shells and plants in moss, and place in a beribboned basket or pot. Experiment with using dyed or decorated eggshells.

FUN WITH FICTIONARY

I generally hate playing games, but recently I was introduced to one that I think is actually fun: fictionary. All you need is a few people and a dictionary. One person starts by opening the dictionary and picking a word that no one knows. Everyone writes down a made-up definition; the dictionary holder writes down the correct definition. Then the dictionary holder collects all definitions and reads them aloud, and everyone votes for the correct one. If someone guesses correctly, he or she gets three points. If no one guesses the correct one, the dictionary holder gets three points. If your wrong definition is chosen, you get one point. Then the dictionary is passed to the next person. The definitions are often quite hilarious; this game offers a chance to be very creative. I once played with friends who made up such believable definitions that I was fooled again and again. I haven't laughed so hard in years.

GIVING BIRDS A HOME

Birds really do like birdhouses, as long as you make them hospitable. Make a birdhouse fit into its surroundings both in color and texture as much as possible (twigs, bark, and unpainted materials are best; birds don't want to feel on display.) Place any house at least six feet off the ground and away from foot and cat traffic. Face it away from the sun, preferably in trees or shrubs. Don't despair if birds don't move in till the second year the house is there; they need time to get used to it.

One easy bird-friendly option is to buy a standard bird-house at a store and hot-glue straw or dried grasses to the roof, creating a natural thatched effect. For more elaborate handmade houses, consult *The Bird Feeder Book* by Thom Boswell and *The Bird House Book* by Bruce Woods and David Schoonmaker (both Lark Books). Lark (800-284-3388) also has a number of birdhouse and bird feeder kits for sale.

SKIN SPRING CLEANING

You can give your skin a great spring cleaning with all-natural products. For oily skin: Mix 1 egg white and 1 tablespoon of oatmeal. Apply in a thin layer to face and neck and leave for 15 to 20 minutes. Egg white contains papain, a natural enzyme that eliminates subcutaneous dirt and oil; the oatmeal is rich in protein and potassium and will give your skin a vital mineral boost. For dry skin: Spread a thin, even layer of honey on face and neck, taking care to avoid eyes. Honey is a natural humectant and traps moisture in the skin.

CUSTOM STATIONERY

With most home computers, you can now create your own stationery. Try typesetting your name and address in different fonts to discover the right image for you. You can also supply your own artwork—do your own simple line drawing or find an image in your computer's image file. Then go to your local quick print shop or copy shop, select the right paper and envelopes, and ask their help in reproduction. Voilà! Unique stationery at a fraction of the cost of store-bought stuff!

SACRED SPOT

You can create an altar or other meaningful contemplative space in just about any nook or cranny of your house—a bookshelf, a ledge above the bathtub, a small table in your bedroom. The point is to pick a place where you will often go so that you can enjoy it. What you decide to place there is, of course, entirely up to you. But whatever you decide on should be something that has meaning for you. It should not be placed on your altar to please your Great-aunt Tilly who gave you that hideous green statue that you really wish some child would conveniently break.

MEXICAN WEDDING COOKIES

Traditional wedding cookies are often served at other festive occasions as well.

½ cup powdered sugar
1 cup butter, softened
1 teaspoon vanilla
2¼ cups flour
¼ teaspoon salt
¾ cup chopped nuts, optional
additional powdered sugar

Cream together the ½ cup sugar, butter, and vanilla in a large bowl. Sift in the flour and salt. Add the nuts, if using. Cover and chill the dough for 2 hours in the refrigerator or 10 minutes in the freezer. Preheat oven to 400°. Roll the dough into 1-inch balls and place on an ungreased cookie sheet. Bake until set, about 10 minutes. While still warm, roll the cookies in powdered sugar. Makes 4 dozen.

BEADING TOGETHER

One great thing to do with kids is to buy an assortment of inexpensive beads (bead and craft stores abound these days) and host a beading party. If you have very young children, you can use dry macaroni (instead of beads that can be popped into mouths) that they can decorate with paint or glitter. You can then help kids string them onto elastic for easy bracelets and necklaces. For older beaders, buy bead thread, beading needles, and clasps to finish off their creations.

EXOTIC LETTUCE MIXES

Are you a fan of those expensive mixed salad greens? You can easily make your own mix by buying lettuce seeds such as oak leaf, black seeded simpson, and red salad bowl as well as arugula, mizuna, watercress, and chicory. In many parts of the country, it is too hot to grow lettuce during the summer. But you can keep them growing even during the summer if you plant new seedlings every few weeks and provide a "roof" made of shade cloth you can buy at any garden supply store. The trick is to harvest when the leaves are very young and tender, otherwise they may become too bitter. When the plants are a few inches high, sheer the tops with scissors; they will grow back quickly, and you'll have salads for weeks. Check out seed catalogs from Vermont Bean (802-273-3400), J. W. Jung Seed (414-326-3121), and Sumway (803-663-9771).

FLORAL SPLASH

It's easy to make your own eau de cologne, with so many essential oils available these days. Here's one version, but feel free to experiment with the essential oils of your choice. If you find this concoction too strong, just dilute it with bottled water. A beautiful antique bottle makes the perfect receptacle.

½ cup 100-proof vodka
sterilized wide-neck glass jar with top
20 drops orange essential oil
10 drops bergamot essential oil
10 drops lemon essential oil
2 drops neroli essential oil
¼ cup bottled water without carbonation
paper coffee filter
sterilized decorative glass bottle
   with top that can hold ¾ cup

Pour the vodka into the wide-mouthed jar and add the essential oils, stirring with a wooden spoon. Put lid on and let stand for 2 days. Add the water and stir. Cover again and let sit for 4 to 6 weeks. Strain through coffee filter and pour into decorative bottle.

TEN-MINUTE FUDGE

Ah, chocolate!

3 squares (1 ounce each) unsweetened chocolate
4 tablespoons butter
4½ cups sifted powdered sugar
⅓ cup instant nonfat dry milk
½ cup light or dark corn syrup
1 tablespoon water
1 teaspoon vanilla
½ cup chopped nuts, optional

Grease an 8-inch square pan. Melt chocolate and butter in the top of a 2-quart double boiler over hot water. Meanwhile, sift together sugar and dry milk in a medium bowl. Stir corn syrup, water, and vanilla extract into chocolate-butter mixture. Stir in sifted sugar and dry milk in two additions. Continue stirring until mixture is well blended and smooth. Remove from heat. Stir in nuts if desired. Pour mixture into pan. Let cool, then cut into squares. Makes 24 2-inch squares.

AROMATIC TRIVET

This kitchen delight will release a fabulous fragrance every time you place a hot pan on it. These trivets are so simple to make, you should consider making some for yourself and for your friends.

20 inches sturdy fabric,
  such as mattress ticking
scissors
needle and thread

stuffing: broken cinnamon
  sticks, cloves, and bay leaves
upholstery needle
cotton string

Cut two 20-to-25-inch pieces of fabric and place right sides together. Pin and stitch the pieces together, leaving an opening large enough for the stuffing to fit through. Trim the seams and turn right side out. Fill with stuffing material and then slip-stitch the opening using the upholstery needle threaded with string. Make four separate stitches in the center of the pad, forming a square, clearing the contents away from the stitch. Finish each with a simple knot. Makes 1 trivet.

HOMEMADE VANILLA EXTRACT

Yes, you can make it yourself, and it is unbelievably easy. If you place the extract in a pretty glass bottle, it makes a lovely little gift.

> 1 vanilla bean
> 1 4-ounce bottle with top
> scant 4 ounces vodka

Split the bean in half, put it in the bottle, and pour in the vodka. Cap and let sit at least one month (the longer, the stronger).

ZEN CENTERPIECE

Truly nothing could be easier than this arrangement; it will foster serenity wherever you place it.

small dark rocks
shallow bowl
3 small floating candles
1 flower such as a gardenia, rose, or hibiscus

Place the rocks in a colander and rinse. Fill the bottom of the bowl with 1 to 2 inches of rocks, depending on the depth of the container—you want to create a rock bottom. Fill with water up to 1 inch from the top rim. Float the candles and gently place the blossom on the water and allow it to float.

HIDE A LOVE NOTE

My friend has had a troubled relationship with her father. But no matter how difficult things between them get, she always remembers that when she was in junior high and high school, after her mother had abandoned the family, her father often put an affectionate note in her backpack, which she would see as she took her books out at school. Those notes not only created joy in those moments but they still do now, years later. Who in your life would be delighted to receive a surprise love note? Tuck one in a child's lunchbox, a spouse's briefcase, under a pillow. You'll give happiness to both of you.

TAKE A DIP
IN THE OCEAN—AT HOME

Have you ever noticed how great you feel after a swim in the ocean? Part of the reason is that the magnesium, zinc, and potassium in sea salt draw out the lactic acid from your muscles, easing tension. You can simulate the effect in a luxurious bath. Pour one cup of salt into the stream of warm water while filling the tub, turn on an ocean CD or tape, light a sea breeze-scented candle, and indulge.

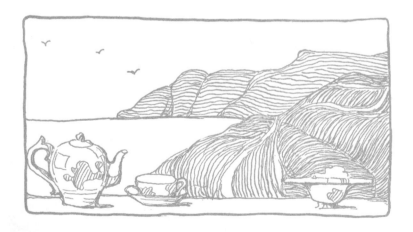

MAKE A MEMORY BOX

Find or buy a box you like and put your favorite things in it. Choose things that feel good because they bring back good memories—the picture of your newborn (he's now twenty-seven), the one earring from the pair your husband bought you while he was on a business trip as a surprise present, the flowers from the day he told you he loved you. As the memories flood back, you will instantly feel happy.

THE ART ROOM

Our family room is a bit different from most people's. It's a corner of a big closed-in porch that we have turned into an art corner. It has a large old table and chairs and a cabinet full of art supplies—paints, glue, papers of all sorts, glitter, Popsicle sticks, pipe cleaners, and dried flowers. Sometimes individually and sometimes together, the three of us—mother, father, and daughter—go in there to create something. We make cards, pictures to hang on the walls, and presents for one another and for other relatives. It's a place where each of us can express our creativity. I love to go in there with my three-year-old and finger-paint, letting the goopy paint squish through my fingers and seeing what color combinations I can create from the three primary colors. Such a simple pleasure!

GIVE A MAY BASKET

When I was a kid, we always made May baskets for all the houses in our neighborhood to celebrate May Day. We would get such a thrill out of hanging them on front door knobs and then ringing the bell and running to a hiding spot, where we'd watch the face of the recipient. May baskets are incredibly easy to make. All you need are some flowers (we always picked the first wildflowers of the season, but store-bought flowers are fine) that you've fashioned into an attractive bouquet tied with a rubber band and placed in a cone basket. To make the cone, take an 8½-by-11-inch piece of construction paper rolled into an ice-cream-cone shape, with the top wider than the bottom. Staple into place and attach a paper handle (a ½-inch-wide strip of construction paper) at the top with staples. Whose day can you brighten with such a gift? Your co-workers? The neighbors? Your daughter?

SWEET SACHET

Here's something middle-school kids can make Mom or Grandmom for Mother's Day.

¼ yard lace	tapestry needle
1 dinner plate	2 yards ¼-inch-wide wired ribbon
disappearing ink marker	2 ounces lavender or potpourri
scissors	2 yards 1-inch-wide ribbon
1 cereal bowl	

Place the lace on a table and lay the dinner plate on top of it. Trace the edge of the plate with the disappearing ink marker. Remove plate and cut around marker to make a circle of lace. Turn the cereal bowl upside down in the center of the lace circle, and trace the edge. Remove bowl. Thread the tapestry needle with the thin ribbon and stitch around the inner circle you have just created. (The size of the stitches doesn't matter.) Tug gently on the ribbon so the lace gathers to make a pocket. When the opening is the size of a silver dollar, pour the lavender or potpourri in until the pouch is full (about the size of a walnut). Tug the ribbon tight, tie in a knot, and cut the ends short. Tie the wide ribbon into a beautiful bow. Repeat until materials are gone. Makes 5 sachets.

HOMEMADE
ALPHA-HYDROXY MASK

Cook half of a diced and peeled apple in ¼ cup of milk until
soft and tender. Mash, then cool to room temperature, and
apply to skin. Thoroughly cleanse with warm water after 15
to 20 minutes.

MORNING WONDER RITUAL

The great cellist Pablo Casals once said, "For the past eighty years, I have started each day in the same manner. It is not a mechanical routine but something essential to my daily life. I go to the piano and I play two preludes and fugues of Bach. I cannot think of doing otherwise. It is a sort of benediction on the house. But that is not its only meaning for me. It is a rediscovery of the world in which I have the joy of being a part. It fills me with awareness of the wonder of life, with a feeling of the incredible marvel of being a human being." What small thing can you do when you wake up in the morning to tap into that sense of marvel? Play a special piece of music? Read something inspirational? For me, it's cuddling in bed with my daughter, looking up at the redwood tree framed in the skylight, and listening to all the birds sing.

WORM FARM

Here's an activity to do with little ones. Search your yard for about ten worms. Fill a gallon glass jar with alternating layers of sand and garden soil until the jar is almost full. Then add compost items such a coffee grounds, banana peels cut into pieces, and old dried leaves. Place the worms on the top and cover with a piece of black cloth. Whenever curiosity strikes, remove the cloth for a few minutes and see what the worms are up to. When interest wanes, return worms to the garden.

DECORATIVE LIGHT SWITCHES

One great activity that families can do together is to decorate the light switches in various rooms of the house. All you need is acrylic paints and small brushes. Take the switch off the wall and paint the design of your choice (mistakes wipe off easily with water). Let dry thoroughly and rescrew into the wall.

WILDFLOWER MEADOW

I don't know about you, but I believe lawns are vastly over-rated. They take a tremendous amount of water and too much labor, and they cause vast quantities of chemicals to be dumped into our water supply. So I decided to dig mine up and plant a wildflower meadow instead. It took some work to get going, but within four weeks I had my first bloom. It was a glorious sight for six months and unlike a lawn, virtually maintenance free. Plus I had an almost end-less supply of cut flowers from late spring to late fall. The tricks are to till the soil in the spring, select a pure wild-flower mix (no grass or vermiculite filler) appropriate to your area, and blend the seed with four times its volume of fine sand so it will disperse evenly. After you've spread it over the dirt, lay down a layer of loose hay to keep the seeds from blowing away. Usually the mixes are a combina-tion of annuals, biannuals, and perennials. To keep the an-nuals going, rough up parts of the soil and reseed just those every year.

GARLIC SOUP

Cultures throughout the world swear by garlic soup as a spring tonic and all-around cure for that under-the-weather feeling. Don't let the huge quantity of garlic scare you off—when cooked it becomes very mellow.

> 4 heads of garlic
> 1 bunch parsley, thyme,
>   or marjoram, tied into a bundle with string
> 1 quart chicken broth, vegetable broth, or water
> juice of 1 lemon or lime
> salt and pepper to taste
> lightly toasted bread or croutons (optional)

Break up the heads of garlic into cloves, and discard the papery membrane, but don't peel the cloves, and place in a 4-quart soup pot with the herbs. Add the broth or water, cover, and bring to a boil. Lower the heat and simmer for about 30 minutes, until garlic is very soft. Strain the soup through the fine disk of a food mill or puree in a blender or food processor, and push through a medium-mesh strainer with the back of a ladle. Add the lemon or lime juice, salt and pepper, and bread or croutons, if desired. Serves 4.

MINTY FACIAL ASTRINGENT

1 tablespoon fresh peppermint
or spearmint
1 cup witch hazel

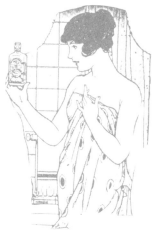

Combine ingredients in a jar with a tight-fitting lid. Steep in cool, dry place for one week, shaking occasionally. Strain and pour liquid into a bottle or spritzer. Use about 1 teaspoon a day on your face. Good for normal and oily skin. Makes about a six-week supply.

HEALTHFUL CLEANING PLEASURES

It's time for a good spring cleaning! How about doing it the nontoxic way?

Baking soda makes a mild cleanser for kitchen and bath fixtures; just sprinkle it straight from the box onto a damp cloth or sponge. Use a few tablespoons dissolved in a quart of water to wash the interiors of refrigerators and freezers, neutralizing odors. Add a tablespoon to coffee pots and vacuum bottles, then fill them with water to freshen them. Still on supermarket shelves, the venerable Bon Ami cleanser is slightly more effective than baking soda and doesn't contain chlorine, phosphates, perfumes, or harsh abrasives. Baking soda with lemon juice will remove soap film in the bathtub and shower. Adding a few teaspoons of vinegar to a quart of water produces a handy glass cleaner, and equal parts of borax and washing soda (sodium carbonate, often labeled as "detergent booster") make an even less pungent solution for the dishwasher. For discolored copper pots, try an early-twentieth-century cleanser: a tablespoon of salt mixed with a half cup of vinegar.

SOAP CARVINGS

You and your kids can have fun making soap carvings as presents and for use at home. Just start with a big cake of soap, a potato peeler, a butter knife, and a nail. Use the peeler to carve a design into the soap, the knife to cut off large areas, and the nail to draw designs.

131

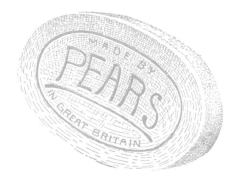

KEEP MEMORIES ALIVE

There are a number of wonderful ways to display photos inexpensively. Here are some ideas to get you started:

- To make photo collages, collect different-sized pictures in frames from yard sales and flea markets. Throw the pictures away. Cut a poster board the size of the frame for the backdrop, then create a collage with snapshots, gluing the pictures to the poster board, and insert into the frame. Think in themes—birthdays, holidays over the years, your daughter's volleyball career, vacation shots of you and your husband.

- Purchase inexpensive clear 8-by-10-inch acrylic box frames and have favorite photos blown up to 8-by-10-inch. Arrange them attractively on the wall.

- Find old window frames without glass. Tack pictures and other mementos on the wall and place the frames over them to create the illusion of looking through a window.

EASY-CARE GARDENING

Too busy to care for a vegetable garden or don't have the room for one? Consider what 100,000 people around the United States do—buy shares in someone else's large garden. All shareholders agree to pay a certain amount per year and, in exchange, get weekly baskets of produce. Depending on where you live, deliveries can be made as often as twenty-two to fifty-two weeks per year.

Like most good ideas, this one has a name—Community Supported Agriculture—and an organization, CSANA. According to CSANA, shares usually cost between $300 and $600 a year. (Many offer discounts for labor; since the work is shared, no one is overburdened, and there's the added bonus of meeting fellow gardeners you might not otherwise know.) For more information about the 600 farms that belong to CSANA, contact them at (413-528-4374) or e-mail csana@bcn.net. Their web address is www.umass.edu/umext/CSA.

PERSONALIZED NAPKIN RINGS

At the craft store, buy a set of clear Lucite napkin rings (the kind with an opening that allows you to put a piece of paper inside). Cut paper to fit inside the rings. Glue pressed flowers in any pleasing arrangement onto the paper, and cover the paper with clear, heavy tape, such as packing tape. Insert the paper into the rings. If you can't find Lucite napkin rings, you can glue pressed flowers directly onto wooden rings, then give them several coats of shellac.

ANIMATED CARDS

This is a pleasure of the e-mail age: sending animated cards to other e-mailers. All kinds of sites offer these now, and many are free; www.cardcentral is a listing of free greeting card sites on the Internet.

You can also look on www.gogreet.com, www.blue-mountain.com, www.postcards.org/postcards, www.comedy-central.com/greetings, and www.marlo.com.

NATURAL HAIR CARE

A simple, effective, old-fashioned hair rinse is good old vinegar, preferably cider vinegar. Mix 2 tablespoons in 2 cups of warm water. Work through hair after shampooing and rinsing, then rinse again with clear water. For light hair, use lemon juice instead of vinegar. This will help restore the natural acid balance of the scalp and get rid of all traces of soap and shampoo. For an all-purpose hair conditioner, combine ¾ cup olive oil, ½ cup honey, and the juice of 1 lemon. Rinse hair with water and towel dry. Work a small amount of conditioner into hair, comb through, and cover with a shower cap or plastic wrap for a half hour. Shampoo and rinse thoroughly. Store remaining conditioner in the refrigerator.

MINIMALIST HOT TUB

Hot tubs can be expensive and time consuming. If you like the idea of bathing outside, consider buying an old-fashioned claw-foot tub (they cost about $100 and fit two people) for outside and run hot and cold water from the house out to it. Because you fill and drain the tub each time (let water trickle into your garden rather than wasting it), you're spared the hassle and expense of chemicals.

HOMEMADE PLAY-DOUGH

This preschool staple is easy to make in batches at home. It's worth keeping an assortment of bottled food coloring for projects like these, even if you don't use them often for cooking.

1 cup salt
1¼ cups water
2 teaspoons vegetable oil
3 cups all-purpose flour (not self-rising)
2 tablespoons cornstarch
Food coloring

In a large bowl, mix salt, water, and vegetable oil. Continue mixing while adding flour and cornstarch. Knead until smooth. If dough seems too sticky, add a little flour. If too dry, add a little water. Divide the dough into several lumps. Add a few drops of food coloring to each lump and knead to mix the color into the dough. Store in airtight containers; the dough will dry out if exposed to air.

ARTISTIC HONOR

Next time you host a party, create a piece of art for the guest of honor. Buy a simple canvas. Divide it into even sections using a pencil and ruler. Go over your pencil lines with permanent colored markers or paint. Provide guests with paints and brushes and have each person decorate a square. Your guest will have a colorful memento of the occasion. This project works well for a variety of occasions: baby showers, housewarmings, high-school graduations, bon voyage parties, and so on.

139

ᘒᘝᘒ

ROOM REFRESHER

If you use a room deodorizer, you don't need to throw it away as the scent begins to wane. Simply put a few drops of your favorite perfume on top of it, and it will continue to scent the air.

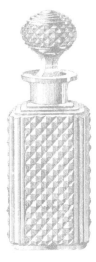

GARDEN JOURNAL

Keeping a garden journal can be wonderfully satisfying. You don't have to limit yourself to the facts—your journal can also be a place to muse, collect quotes, and keep in touch with nature's wisdom. The key is to recognize that it can be a visual record as well as a written one—dry and paste the first sweet pea your son grew; the photos of your orchid cactus in bloom; a smattering of fall leaves on the day you found out you were pregnant, surrounded by the poem your husband wrote for the occasion; sketch the color of the sky on a memorable winter day. Workshop leader Barry Hopkins, who calls these Earthbound Journals, suggests you start with a blank, hardcover artist sketchbook, at least 7½ by 8½, an Exacto knife for cutting, watercolors for borders, Craypas for flowers, aerosol glue for pasting, and fixative to keep pencils and Craypas from smudging.

Make your own cover for your journal—you can use old bits of a special shirt, for example. If you have an electric drill, drill through the book to create a ribbon or rawhide fastener. Follow your own creativity where it leads you and imbue the book with the memories of the garden.

PUBLIC GARDENING

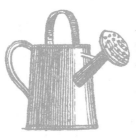

Are you longing for a garden but have no place for one? Take advantage of the variety of places that have gardens: zoos, public parks, cemeteries, college campuses, garden club tours, nurseries and garden centers, or a friend's house. These days, you can also find community gardens and gardening coops in which you can get your hands dirty. Call your parks and recreation department. (All of the above are also great places to get ideas if you do have a garden.)

STEAMING CLEAN

You don't need to go to a spa or to buy any fancy equipment to enjoy a facial steam. All you need is a large pot of boiling water, a sturdy table, a handful of herbs, and a bath towel. Bring a large pot of water to a boil. Remove from heat and add a handful each of whole sage leaves, whole peppermint leaves, and chamomile flowers. Carry the pot over to the table along with the bath towel and sit down in front of the pot. Drape the towel over your head and shoulders so that you and the pot are under the towel, being sure to keep your face at least a foot away from the pot. Breathe slowly and deeply through the nose, lifting the towel to get fresh air as needed. Stay under the towel tent for 5 to 10 minutes. When you're done, moisturize your face with a good lotion. This practice is not recommended if you have extremely dry skin, heart trouble, asthma, or other breathing problems.

FLOWER GREETING CARDS

Place pressed flowers that you've made or bought in a pattern you like on the front of blank cards or on stiff artists' paper available at craft or variety stores. Attach them to the paper with a dab of glue. Peel an appropriate amount of transparent, self-stick plastic film (like contact paper) from the roll and carefully place on top of the flowers, pressing from the center to the edge to eliminate air bubbles. Trim the edge of the plastic to match the card or paper. You can then send them to your friends for Christmas, Hanukkah, birthdays, Valentine's Day, or for no reason at all. Bookmarks can be made in exactly the same way—just cut the paper to an appropriate size.

DEEP BREATH

If you run yourself ragged rushing through the day and seem not to be able to find a time to slow down, take a tip from Vietnamese Buddhist monk Thich Nhat Hahn, who recommends that each time the telephone rings, you notice three breaths before you answer. He suggests it as a way to become aware of the present moment, but it is also fabulous for coming back into your body and reducing tension. The more the phone rings, the more relaxed and present you will be!

SPROUTS IN A JAR

Raw sprouts are a wonderful source of vitamins. Any beans—soy, fava, lima, pinto, garbanzo—can be sprouted, as can alfalfa, sunflower, peas, lentils, and many other seeds. Just be sure never to try potatoes or tomatoes—the sprouts are poisonous. And don't sprout seeds that have been sold for garden planting; they've probably been treated with a fungicide. Untreated seeds are available at health food stores.

> 2 tablespoons alfalfa seeds
> 1 wide-mouth quart jar
> water
> cheesecloth
> rubber band

Place the seeds in the bottom of the jar and fill the jar with water. Put cheesecloth over the top and secure with a rubber band. Store in a warm, dark place, such as a kitchen cupboard. Two or three times a day take the jar out, empty the water, and add new water. The sprouts will be ready in 4 to 5 days and will keep up to a week in the refrigerator. Makes 1 quart.

GIVE YOURSELF A NIGHT OUT

My husband gets together with a group of five other guys once a month to play poker. These guys have been playing together for fifteen years. They take turns making dinner and hosting the event, and my husband never makes it home before 2:00 A.M. I used to turn my nose up at these nights out, but I've come to see that they provide a chance for the friends not only to have fun but to keep connected to one another. They've been there for marriages, births, work changes, breakups, and so on. But the main point is to have fun, and what's wrong with that? Sometimes we all need to go out, stay up late, and kick up our heels. When was the last time you did something like that?

NATURAL
BREATH FRESHENER

Pass around a bowl of mint sprigs after dinner to help everyone deal with the bad breath brought on by eating lots of garlic or onions.

BLOOMING CARD

Some creative person figured out how to plant seeds inside paper, and now a variety of places offer wonderful cards and notepaper that can be written on, mailed, and then planted either inside or out by your lucky letter recipient. Some of best ones I've seen are done by the Santa Fe Farmer's Market Cooperative Store and are handmade from organic and recycled materials and studded with flowers, herbs, and vegetable seeds. The paper disintegrates when you plant it, and the seeds blossom into evidence of your feelings. Available from Seeds of Change; just call (888-762-7333).

HOMEMADE HERBAL TEAS

It's easy to grow and make your own herbal teas, according to the folks at Yamagami's Nursery in Cupertino, California, who write that one way to start is to grow lemon verbena, lemongrass, spearmint, and peppermint. Lemon verbena is easy to grow in full sun to part shade. Prune it frequently to keep it bushy. Widely used in Asian cuisine, lemongrass is a very fragrant clump grass that grows two to three inches tall and likes full sun. Spearmint and peppermint like moist semishady areas; prune them frequently to keep them low, and beware—they can be invasive so you might want to grow them in containers.

You can throw a small handful of any or all of these fresh herbs into black tea before steeping—just be sure to wash them well beforehand. Or you can dry them and experiment with a variety of combinations and additions, including carefully washed rose petals and hips, chamomile buds or leaves, or lemon or orange slices. A good basic caffeine-free recipe is 3 tablespoons dried lemon verbena, 4 tablespoons dried lemongrass, 1 tablespoon dried spearmint, and 1 tablespoon dried peppermint. Simply crumble dried herbs together, steep in 4 cups of boiling water for 5 minutes and strain. Delicious either hot or iced.

BIRD HAVEN

When the birds have begun to build their nests, that's the
time to be generous with your lint after cleaning the screen
in your dryer. Instead of throwing the lint away, put it out
on a porch railing or even a branch of a tree. The birds will
use it to line their homes.

151

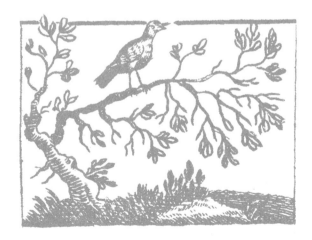

INSTANT ROOM MAKEOVER

If you are tired of the way your living room or bedroom looks, do an instant makeover by revitalizing old throw pillows. Place a pillow kitty-corner on top of a pretty scarf or bandanna. Bring opposing corners of the scarf or bandanna together and tie them in a knot. Do the same with the other corners. Now you have a new, colorful look for your home.

152

CANDLE FIRE

As the weather begins to warm and you no longer use the fireplace, evoke the romance and beauty of a fire by placing four or five pillar candles inside it. The soft light they give off will compensate for the loss of the roaring fire.

153

AROMATHERAPY,
AU NATUREL

154

Every time you pass a lilac bush or some iris or daffodils in flower, take the time to bury your face in the bloom. Lilacs have a sweet and heady scent, and irises are musky and erotic. Close your eyes, breathe deeply, and imagine the fragrance passing through your body.

REFLECTED GLORY

Martha Stewart is renowned for making beautiful things that are often complicated to do. However, sometimes she has an idea that is simplicity itself. One such suggestion we recently saw is to line the edges of a garden path with pure white stones, pebbles, and shells. That way, at nightfall, "they'll reflect the moonlight, showing you the way."

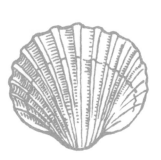

CANDIED FLOWERS

These delectable treats are easy to create; use them on top of ice cream or cakes. Pick the flowers fresh in the early morning.

> violet blossoms
> rose petals
> 1 or 2 egg whites, depending on
>   how many flowers you use
> superfine sugar, to taste

Gently wash flowers and pat dry with a clean towel. Beat the egg whites in a small bowl. Pour the sugar into another bowl. Carefully dip the flowers into the egg whites, then roll in sugar, being sure to cover all sides. Set flowers on a cookie sheet and allow to dry in a warm place. Store in a flat container with waxed paper between layers. The flowers will last for several days.

SURPRISE SOMEONE

My stepdaughter recently went to Europe. Just before she left, while she was in the bathroom, I snuck $100 into her backpack with a card saying it was "splurge" money. I had such fun thinking of the idea, finding the perfect hiding place, trying not to get caught. It was so enjoyable that it didn't even matter to me if she appreciated the gesture or not! (She did! She found the treat days later, when rooting around in her pack.) Put a little lift in your life and surprise someone you know.

TOPIARY TRICKS

If you are attracted to the topiaries you see at botanical gardens, you might want to try growing one of your own. First you need a frame. Some home and garden stores are now carrying them, but you can also get them from Cliff Finch Zoo (209-822-2315), Topiaries Unlimited (802-823-5536), and Topiary Inc. (write for their catalogue: 41 Bering St., Tampa FL 33606).

Then pick a plant to cover it with. Think about where the topiary will be—in the sun or shade? Is it small enough to be brought inside in winter or must the plant be winter hardy? Then think of the plant itself—does it shear nicely? (To help it keep its shape, you must give it a haircut regularly.) Is the leaf size in proportion to the frame, and will the texture give you your desired effect? Good topiary plants include ivy, star jasmine, purple bell vine, Japanese boxwood, pyracantha, rosemary, lavender, and compact myrtle.

RESTORATIVE BATH

This bath a great pick-me-up.

cotton bath bag or piece of cheesecloth
2 tablespoons grated fresh ginger
1 ounce fresh rosemary
20 drops rosemary oil
20 drops lavender oil
1 cup rose water

Place the fresh ginger and rosemary in a cotton bath bag, or bundle in a 1-foot square piece of unused cheesecloth. Tie it closed. Place the bag under the bathtub spigot and run under hot water. Add oils and rose water to the bathtub, swirling with your hand to combine. The bath bag makes an excellent scrubber and exfoliator, and the ginger and rosemary will leave skin pleasantly tingling and feeling revived.

RECORD A NEW MESSAGE

I love it when I call two particular acquaintances of mine, because they have such interesting outgoing messages on their answering machine. One recites her favorite poem of the moment; the other is just incredibly exuberant about what she's doing and why she isn't there to take your call, and she finishes with: "You can leave offers to take me to dinner, or other delicious suggestions at the sound of the beep." Spread some joy to your callers—tell a joke, offer an inspiring quotation, say whatever will make you smile when you record it and your friends smile when they call.

HERBAL SKIN CLEANERS

Many dried herbs are good for the skin. Here are the best herbs for various purposes and skin types:

relaxing: chamomile, lavender, St. John's wort

softening: chamomile, lavender, rose, St. John's wort

cleansing: arnica, calendula, chamomile, comfrey, elderflower, lavender, nettle, peppermint, rosemary, yarrow

soothing: arnica, calendula, chamomile, elderflower, green tea, lavender, rose, witch hazel

stimulating: gingko bilboa, nettle, peppermint, rosemary

nourishing: comfrey, ginkgo biloba, ginseng, St. John's wort

rejuvenating: arnica, calendula, chamomile, comfrey, green tea, ginkgo biloba, ginseng, lavender, rosemary

Decide what kind of herbal mixture you need for your face. Then soak 1 heaping teaspoon of an herb or blend in a cup of whole, unpasteurized milk. Store the mixture in the refrigerator for a few hours, then strain and save milk. To use, rinse your face in warm water, and use cotton balls to apply the milk to face, avoiding eyes. Rinse with warm water and then with cool.

GET A MAKEOVER

This is another feel-good, absolutely free simple pleasure. Just go to any large department store and cruise the makeup counters. Choose someone to make you over. Perhaps you'll end up liking how you look so much that you buy some skin and beauty products. But you can have fun playing whether or not you buy anything. (I also love to go to the wig section and see how I'd look in various hair colors and styles; I make a hideous blonde!)

FLOWER SALADS

Several common flowers are edible—and add color and surprise to an ordinary green salad. Not all flowers are edible, though, so make sure the ones you choose are, and wash and dry thoroughly them before using. Common edibles include nasturtiums, roses, borage, marigolds, squash flowers, and violets.

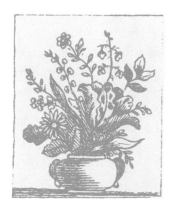

VASEFUL OF JOY

One of the little things I regularly take true delight in is flower arranging. Although I am not good with my hands (my sister used to leave the house in fear when I was learning to sew in junior high), I do get the urge to make something beautiful, and over the years I have discovered that flower arranging is my creative medium. I don't spend a lot of money—I don't have fancy vases, and I don't buy exotic blooms. I work from whatever is blooming in my garden or selling for a few dollars at the flower stand. At holidays I may splurge a bit, but I usually use just a few homegrown roses or roadside poppies or a sprig of holly from the tree in my yard. I have never read a book about the principles of flower arranging and don't spend too much time on it— maybe five minutes at the most. For me, the joy comes from how easy it is to make something pleasing: selecting an old yellow mustard jar, filling it with blue cornflowers, and placing it on the kitchen table. Ongoing beauty, meal after meal, in only a few minutes!

SUN TEA

Sun tea is great because it has a mellower flavor than brewed tea. Drop four tea bags in a quart pitcher of water (the pitcher must be glass). Cover to keep out bugs, and put the pitcher outside in the full sun. After a few hours, when the sun is really hot and you are too, remove the tea bags. Add ice and serve. For a variation, use peach tea. When the tea is ready, cut up a chilled peach into bite-sized pieces and add to the tea. Serve immediately for a one-of-a-kind refresher.

TIME FOR THYME

Grow a yard of woolly thyme instead of grass. Not only is it easier to care for and (virtually) never needs watering, it will hold the heat of the day's sun and fill your yard with a singularly pleasing smell. At the very least, try it between the stones or bricks of your front walk or garden path. Every time you walk across it, the smell will waft up. (And you can use it in any recipe that calls for thyme.)

FABULOUS FOOT RUB

If a foot rub is your idea of a good time, try doing one with peppermint foot lotion. Many people swear by it as the only curative after a long walk or a hard day of work (or of shopping!). The Body Shop sells a superior foot lotion. You can also make your own by adding 1 tablespoon of peppermint oil to 6 ounces of unscented lotion. Or try this therapeutic indulgence, courtesy of the Fredericksburg Herb Farm in Fredericksburg, Texas: grate approximately 1 cup of fresh ginger. Squeeze gently and add, along with a few drops of olive oil, to a foot basin or tub filled with hot water. Cover the bowl with a cloth or towel to preserve the heat, and soak for fifteen minutes. Then dry your feet and slip into a pair of warm socks.

MAKE YOUR OWN PERFUME

With essential oils, you can create your own perfume, based on your mood at the time. All you need is an eye-dropper and a variety of oils. Kimberley D. Wheat, buyer for Bare Escentuals, offers her favorite secret recipe which she calls "Little Black Dress": 2 drops ylang-ylang, 1 drop patchouli, and 1 drop bergamot added to 1 teaspoon jojoba oil. "Apply to pulse points!" Remember, essential oils are to be used only externally. Be sure not to ingest them; they can be toxic or even fatal. Be sure to keep them out of the reach of children, and test each one on a spot on your arm before you use them liberally in baths or as perfumes.

OLD-FASHIONED GAMES

School is out. When the kids have been cooped up in the house too long playing Nintendo and watching TV and have steam to let off, why not suggest that they round up the neighbor kids and try a batch of the games that were popular in previous generations? You'll recognize them: leap frog, hopscotch, king of the hill, duck, duck goose, red light, Mother may I, Simon says, marbles, and jacks. Who says fun has to come in a box and cost $50 or more? Maybe they will even entice you to join them in a trip down memory lane.

169

KID-SAFE AROMATHERAPY

With the popularity of aromatherapy these days, many parents are wondering if it's safe for children. Essential oils in particular can be quite strong, so here are a few guidelines:

1. Always dilute essential oils before applying to children's sensitive skin. You can use oils such as sweet almond, grapeseed, or jojoba for massages or skin care and liquid castile soap for shower products. But never put essential oils directly onto a child's skin.

2. Shake well before using, because the oils have a tendency to separate.

3. Keep all essential oils out of the reach of children. The same goes for diffusers; small children have been known to drink the oils in them.

If you want to be sure the products you're using are safe for kids, try getting a catalogue from Aromatherapy for Kids (800-955-8353) or from Star Power Essentials (800-457-0904).

BLOW BUBBLES

This pleasure requires a bit of money—89 cents or so! Buy an eight-ounce bottle of bubbles, find a small child or receptive adult and a good spot outside, and let yourself go. I guarantee you'll have a good time. Watch how the wind carries the bubbles hither and yon. Blow a few to the other person and see if she can catch them. Allow yourself the indulgence of being two years old again, if only for fifteen minutes.

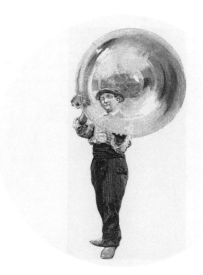

SIMPLE PLEASURES OF SUMMER

Today is the first day of summer. Hurrah! Maybe it's because of our experience of summer vacation as kids, but summer is the season that makes most of us the happiest. Eating outdoors, flowers bursting in yards, swimming, boating, water-skiing, sailing, fresh cherries and nectarines! What are the little things that give you pleasure in the summer? Make a list, and be sure to fit them all in this year.

CELEBRATE THE SOLSTICE

I love the sun, and so it is natural for me to celebrate the summer solstice, the longest day of the year, with a barbecue bash on my deck for all my friends. I always serve sangria to the adults and lemonade to the kids, ask everyone to bring their own food to barbecue, make a big vat of potato salad, and voilà: instant celebration. We feast and laugh—kids and grownups alike—play silly games like red rover and blind man's bluff, and we have a grand old time enjoying the first day of summer.

FLOWER TIEBACKS

I love the romantic look of lace curtains in my bedroom. Recently I came across a wonderful rose tieback that is quite easy to make and looks great against the lacy fabric. They're delicate, so once they are on the curtains try to avoid taking them on and off all the time.

½-inch satin ribbon
moss
small dried roses

Tie a length of ribbon around the curtain you want to tie back and cut to correct length. Mark the area that covers the front with two straight pins, one on either end. Glue small pieces of moss to the area between the two pins. Glue roses attractively into the moss. With scissors, trim away any unsightly moss. Tie onto curtain. Makes 1 tieback.

LAVENDER LOTION

For a beautiful gift, try buying some beautiful bottles with stoppers and decorate them with dried lavender sprigs and a raffia bow. These are so easy, you can make lots to give away!

8 ounces unscented body lotion
30 drops lemon essential oil
30 drops lavender essential oil

Pour the lotion into a glass bowl and add the essential oils. Mix well. Using a funnel, fill container of choice, seal, and decorate. Makes 8 ounces.

FLOWER LIGHTS

Here's an easy way to decorate your backyard for a summertime evening get-together—or just for yourself.

silk flowers
one strand of small white
  indoor-outdoor Christmas lights
½-inch-wide white or gold ribbon
plastic or silk green leaves
hot glue

Pull apart the silk flowers and discard the stem. Take the light strand and push a light through the center of one flower. Hot-glue the ribbon to one end and begin wrapping the strand of lights. As you wrap, hot-glue the leaf stem to the chord and cover the leaf stems with the ribbon.

SAND LAMPS

When the weather starts to turn warm and you want to hold an evening garden party, consider this easy-to-make lighting. Simply buy some beautiful terra-cotta pots (or use the ones your plants have grown out of, but make sure they are terra-cotta, not plastic). Make a plug of masking tape over the drain hole, fill the pot with sand, and insert a fat candle. Shield the candle from the wind with hurricane-lamp chimneys, available at home improvement and import stores such as Pier 1and Cost Plus.

HOMEMADE WATER SLIDE

For a special summer treat, you can create your very own water slide. All you need is a patch of lawn, a large sheet of plastic, rocks, a garden hose, and a lawn sprinkler. Simply spread the plastic on the lawn and weigh the edges down with rocks. Hook the sprinkler up to the hose and thoroughly wet the plastic. Then turn the kids loose to slip and slide, periodically wetting down the plastic to keep it slippery.

DAISY CHAINS

I grew up next to a field where all sorts of wildflowers bloomed—daisies and black-eyed Susans, buttercups and Queen Anne's lace. One of my favorite things to do on lazy summer afternoons was to collect daisies and make a chain. Sometimes I would wear the chain in my hair, sometimes festoon the headboard in my bedroom, sometimes offer it as a present to my mother. I still remember how to make one. The trick is to cut the daisies with long (one foot) stems. You start with three blooms on a flat surface—the ground is just fine—staggered at various heights. Braid these together. Then add a fourth daisy to the center of the three and brain into the chain. Continue as long as you have daisies, time, or patience. Tie off the end with a knot.

BARBEQUED BANANAS

Meat and vegetables are not the only barbeque candidates!

4 bananas
lemon juice to taste
dark brown sugar to taste
butter

Peel bananas. Brush each with lemon juice, sprinkle with sugar, and dot with butter. Wrap tightly in double thick aluminum foil and grill for about 15 minutes, turning frequently. Remove from grill and remove foil. Serves 4.

INDULGE IN
CREATURE COMFORTS

Why do we deny ourselves so many creature comforts? I never buy the peach tea I love because it costs slightly more than regular tea. I can afford it, but I feel guilty indulging myself. How silly—my happiness is worth $1 more a week! Wear that special pair of earrings, your favorite shirt, the perfume you save for special occasions. Today's special occasion is your own pleasure.

THE PLEASURE OF SOUND

If you want a more sophisticated sound for your garden than wind chimes normally offer, consider garden bells. They are a set of cup-shaped metal bells on wires that come with a base. Like chimes, they peal when blown by the breeze. Unlike chimes, however, the tones change when they are filled with rain, and their sound can be adjusted by bending the wires. Call Woodstock Percussion at 800-422-4463.

FAMILY SLUMBER PARTY

When my in-laws are visiting, we sometimes prepare a late-night snack (such as ice cream with fruit sauce), change into pajamas, open the futon in the family room, bring plenty of extra blankets, spread out on sofas and mattresses, and tell stories. We stay up late, then fall asleep all together. It is then that I feel most like a part of their big, warm-hearted family.

"STAINED-GLASS" VOTIVES

Here's a kid activity that's worth sharing.

small baby food jars
tissue paper, different colors
liquid starch
ribbon
tea candles

Wash baby food jars thoroughly and take off the labels. Cut different colors of tissue paper into small squares. Pour liquid starch in a spray bottle; spray starch on a jar and then apply squares of tissue paper all over the outside of the jar until it's completely covered. Let dry. Tie a ribbon around the neck of the jar, and place a tea light candle inside. When the light shines through, it is quite lovely.

CARAMEL APPLES

These make an incredibly wonderful barbeque treat at a Fourth of July party—one that all your friends must make for themselves! Be careful to let them cool completely before eating—caramel has a tendency to cool slowly.

4 medium apples
small bowl melted butter
small bowl brown sugar
finely chopped peanuts (optional)

Place each apple on a shish-kebab skewer. Hold it over the coals, turning frequently, until the skin can be pulled off. Without removing it from the skewer, peel, dip apple in butter, then in brown sugar, covering completely. Hold skewer over grill and slowly turn until sugar becomes caramelized. Dip in peanuts if desired, and cool completely. Serves 4.

PRODUCE FOR APARTMENT DWELLERS

If you have no space or time for a garden (or are plagued by critters eating your goodies before you get to them), try creating hanging vegetable baskets. According to experts, almost anything can be grown in a basket, but be sure to get compact growing varieties of the vegetables you want. Buy 14-inch diameter wire baskets (16-inch for zucchini or watermelons). It's best to grow one type of vegetable per basket, although a variety of lettuces or herbs will work well together.

Line basket with sphagnum moss and fill with potting soil. Plant seedlings rather than seeds, and hang the baskets outdoors from patios or rafters, where they will get at least four hours of afternoon sun. Avoid over watering seedlings, but once they become established you do need to feed and water frequently; on the hottest days, they may even need to be watered twice. Once seedlings are three weeks old, fertilize every three weeks with an all-purpose soluble fertilizer, but never feed unless the soil is damp.

ELDERFLOWER SKIN REFRESHER

If you live in an area where elderflowers grow, here's a recipe for an old-fashioned skin tonic. This makes a great gift when packaged in a beautiful glass bottle decorated with an old botanical illustration of an elderflower. Be sure to include storage instructions.

50 elderflower heads, washed in cold water
1 quart jar, sterilized
2½ cups water
5 tablespoons vodka
cheesecloth
decorative glass bottles with lids

Remove petals from heads, making sure not to bruise the flowers; do not include stems. Place petals in quart jar. Boil water and pour over flowers. Let stand for 30 minutes and add vodka. Cover and let stand on counter for 24 hours. Pour liquid through cheesecloth into glass bottles and cap. Store in refrigerator until used. Then keep in cool, dry, dark place like a cabinet and use within one month. Makes 3 cups.

MINT FOOT SCRUB

1 cup unflavored yogurt
1 cup kosher or rock salt
¾ cup mint leaves

Combine ingredients and apply the mixture to your feet. Use a damp washcloth to gently scrub rough spots. Rinse feet and apply a thick lotion or some petroleum jelly.

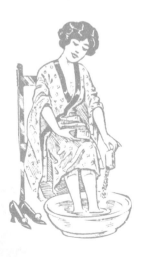

GARDENING SOAP

Ever wonder what to do with all those slivers of soap? I slip them into the leg of an old pair of pantyhose, clip the leg off, and tie it to my spigot outside. Now I have a convenient place to wash my hands after gardening.

COLORFUL DRIED HERBS

When you dry your own herbs, they don't have to turn black or brown. Try this simple trick: put freshly cut herbs that have been washed and well dried into a paper lunch bag, close the bag with a clothespin, and punch four holes in different places in the bag with a fork. Put the bag in the refrigerator. Each morning when you first open the fridge, give the bag a shake and turn it over. When the herbs are completely dry, store in a container until ready to use. Your parsley, chives, and so on will be bright green all year long!

BUILD A SAND CASTLE

What fun! All you really need to make a sand castle is a few buckets, some shovels and trowels, and some spoons. You'll attract plenty of young helpers. Pick a flat spot where the tide is going out. And don't forget the sunscreen! If you want to go high tech, check out www.sandsculpture.com, where professional sand sculptors share their secrets.

SIMPLE SUMMER REFRESHERS

Freeze little slices of lemon or lime into your ice cubes for a pretty and refreshing touch in ice tea or other cold drinks. You can also freeze orange or cranberry juice into ice cubes to add sparkle to lemon-lime soda.

192

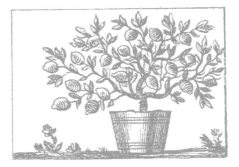

OUTDOOR SHOWERS

One of the best things my mother ever did when we kids were little was to introduce us to outdoor showers. It would be a hot sticky summer day in New England, and suddenly a rainstorm would come up. She would dress us in our bathing suits and let us run outside. The best part was standing under the drain spout and letting the water beat down on our heads. The sense of freedom and excitement from doing something new, the relief from the heat and humidity, the peculiar smell of water meeting superheated asphalt—I can still remember it vividly forty years later.

COOL AND SOOTHING

When the weather is hot and sticky, refrigerate your facial toner, freshener, astringent, or aftershave. It will be as cool as the advertisements in the glossy magazines promise.

194

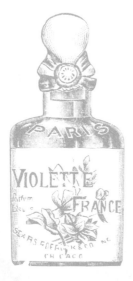

HERBAL AND FLORAL WATERS

To evoke the simplicity of gentler times, do as nineteenth-century women did and make yourself fresh herbal or floral water. You can use these delightfully fragranced waters in many ways. Use them as you would a body splash or toilet water, place them in a bowl to scent your home, or put them in an atomizer and use them to infuse your home or body with sweet fragrance.

> 3 cups distilled water
> ¼ cup of vodka (unlike rubbing alcohols, vodka will not add its own scent to the mixture)
> 1 ounce dried flowers, or 8 to 10 drops of essential oil (this is a guide only; use more or less to your taste)

Measure the water into a bottle, add the vodka, then mix in the flowers, herbs, or oils. Let the mixture stand, covered, in a dark, cool place for seven days. You can leave the herbs or flowers in if you want, or if they aren't as attractive as when they were you started (which is often the case), simply strain them out.

HOMEMADE VANILLA ICE CREAM

When the French novelist Stendhal first tasted ice cream, he declared, "What a pity this isn't a sin!" Judge for yourself.

3 cups half-and-half
¾ cup sugar
6 egg yolks
2 teaspoons vanilla extract

In a heavy saucepan, bring the half-and-half to a simmer over medium heat. In a heatproof bowl, whisk together the sugar and egg yolks until well blended. Gradually pour the hot half-and-half into the egg mixture, whisking continually. Return mixture to saucepan and cook over medium-low heat, stirring with a wooden spoon, until the custard is thick enough to coat a spoon, about 5 minutes.

Pour the custard through a strainer into a clean bowl and refrigerate until cold. Transfer the custard to an ice cream freezer and follow manufacturer's instructions for freezing. If possible, let stand 2 or 3 hours before serving. Makes about 5 cups.

CHILL OUT

Here's a hot-weather tip from the character played by Marilyn Monroe in the movie version of *The Seven Year Itch*, George Axelrod's Broadway comedy. She chilled her underwear in the refrigerator before getting dressed!

197

HOMEMADE LEIS

You can easily string your own leis, using a variety of flowers. Some of the best are tuberose, rose (use buds, not open flowers), carnations, and asters. You will need a long (1 to 2 inches) sewing needle and unscented dental floss. Measure a length of the floss around your neck; leis are most comfortable when they reach nearly to your waist. String a bead or make a large knot in one end of the floss. Trim each flower so that only the blossom remains; then, starting from the stem end, insert the needle and push through the center of the blossom and out the other end. (You may be more comfortable wearing a thimble.) Continue until the string is full, with ¼ inch remaining to be tied off (you will probably need more flowers than you think!). Leis can also be made with paper flowers or candy, even dry cereal! They make excellent centerpieces too.

BASIL, MINT, AND ROSE HIP TEA

Some folks swear by hot tea in hot weather as a cool down technique.

12 ounces water
2 tablespoons chopped fresh spearmint
2 tablespoons chopped fresh basil
2 rose hip teabags
honey or sugar to taste (optional)

Place the water, spearmint, and basil in a nonreactive pan. Cover and bring the water to a rolling boil. Remove lid, stir, then add the teabags. Steep, covered, for 3 minutes. Strain tea into 2 warmed cups. Sweeten with honey or sugar, if desired. Serves 2.

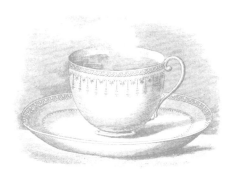

PRESSED FLOWERS

Making pressed flowers is incredibly easy. It requires no special equipment and costs absolutely nothing. Here's how: when your new telephone book comes, save the old one and put it somewhere where you won't lose it. Find a meadow and collect small bouquets of wildflowers. Lay them flat in different parts of the phone book. Place a small boulder, or anything else that's heavy and not likely to take off, on top of the phone book. Let sit for a few months.

200

SANDWICH MASK

Here's a great cool-down for a hot day.

½ cup mayonnaise
1 large tomato
1 medium-sized cucumber, chopped
½ large avocado, mashed

Purée the ingredients in a blender or mixer until smooth. Apply to skin and allow to dry. Rinse well and follow with a light toner and moisturizer.

SEED-SPITTING CONTEST

Wait for a really hot day and wear an old T-shirt. Then sit outside with a friend, take a mouthful of watermelon and spit the seeds as far as you can. For an added bonus, let the juice dribble down your chin and chest.

TOUCH-ME MASSAGE OIL

4 ounces sweet almond oil
½ teaspoon of your favorite essential oil

Blend the oils well in a bowl and then pour into a small decorative glass bottle with a top. Add a beautiful ribbon, and you have a wonderful gift. Be sure to shake oils well before using.

203

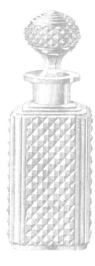

ROCK CANDY

Remember this old-fashioned candy? Making it is a great kid-friendly cooking project.

1 cup sugar
1 cup water
1 teaspoon vanilla, peppermint,
   or other flavoring, optional
wooden skewers about 3 inches long
small wide-necked glass bottles or jars
   (like the kind apple juice comes in)
food coloring
aluminum foil

Boil water and sugar until sugar is completely dissolved. Add flavoring if desired. Pour into bottles or jars and add food coloring, one color per jar, stirring with wooden skewer. Cover the jar top with foil, then poke a wooden skewer through the foil into each jar. Let sit until sugar water has cooled and crystals have formed. Voilà—rock candy. Makes 1 cup; quantity varies depending on number of jars.

LEGACY OF TREES

Our family has decided to plant three trees, representing our three family members, in each of the fifty states. The places we're picking contain either our last name or one of our first names. We're doing it because we believe planting trees is a way to help protect nature, to beautify the landscape, and to provide habitat for birds and animals. So far we've been to twenty states and have been received graciously in each town we've visited. We generally find a family that is willing to have us plant a tree in their yard, but we've also done a few street trees.

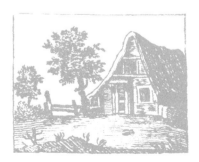

PRESSED-FLOWER PAPERWEIGHTS

These paperweights are truly a simple pleasure. Make some pressed flowers and buy a hollow glass mold at a craft store. Trace the bottom of the mold onto a piece of mat board. Cut out the mat, arrange the pressed flowers on it, then glue flowers in place. Hot-glue the glass mold to the mat; when dry, glue a circle of felt to the bottom.

GENUINE CHOCOLATE MALT

If you prefer vanilla, omit the chocolate syrup. Either way,
be sure your malted milk powder is not chocolate flavored.

4 scoops vanilla ice cream
1½ cups milk
3 tablespoons chocolate syrup
1 teaspoon vanilla extract
2 tablespoons malted milk powder

Whip up all ingredients in blender. Serves 1.

SOUND-SLEEP SUGGESTIONS

Doesn't getting lots of sleep feel great? Experts say we are a sleep-deprived nation and that we need between seven and eight hours of sleep a night, no matter how absorbed we are in that new novel or late-night talk show. Shorten sleeping time, and we lose that most valuable period just before we awaken, when our bodies recharge to deal with stress.

Here's some common advice: get to bed a half hour earlier than usual and, after a few weeks, add another half hour. Ease toward bedtime with quiet activities such as reading, stretching, and meditation. Don't drink caffeine in the evening, and don't smoke or drink alcohol before bedtime. To deal with continual insomnia, one study by a clinical psychologist has come up with dramatically reverse advice: spend less time in bed to cut down on the frustration of lying awake. Forced to stay awake until, say, 1:00 A.M., insomniacs drop off to sleep more easily. When they were able to sleep soundly during those limited hours, they gradually extended their time in bed. One more intriguing idea—use the bedroom exclusively for sleep and sex.

PEPPY POPPIES

To prolong the life of poppies and other sap-filled flowers such as hibiscus, hollyhocks, clematis, and hellebores, try this trick before you arrange them. Cut the stems to the desired length then hold them over a match flame for a few seconds to sear the stems. This will seal the stems and keep the sap from draining out, extending the life of your bouquet.

EASY REFRESHER

I don't know whether I'm so excited about this refresher because it's so fabulous (which I believe it is) or because I invented a beauty product on my own. Last summer, when it was quite hot, I got it into my mind (I guess because I read that green tea is good for the skin) to mix equal parts cooled green tea and water in a spray bottle. I sprayed it all over my face—it felt and smelled wonderful. I'm hooked on the stuff now.

HATFUL OF BEAUTY

For a summer garden party, beautify your old straw hat with a ribbon of fresh flowers. All you need besides the hat is raffia, scissors, and some flowers. Try flowers that will last a long time out of water—sunflowers, statice, yarrow, chrysanthemums, carnations, and daisies are best, as are sturdy greens like sword ferns. Cut the greens and flowers with long enough stems to bundle. Separate each kind and create hand-sized bunches of each. Set aside. Cut several strands of raffia long enough not only to go around the hat's crown but also to wrap around the flower bundles. Knot the strands together at one end. Starting 6 inches from the knotted end, twist the raffia around the stems of one bunch of flowers several times. Lay the next bunch down as far apart from the previous bunch as you like, and repeat the wrapping process Continue down the length of raffia until you have a garland long enough to go around the hat. Place the garland on the hat and tie the two ends of raffia together; tuck any loose raffia under the flowers. To keep fresh for several days, store hat in the refrigerator in a plastic bag.

CONFETTI EGGS

This is a fun project, especially for kids. But be sure to crack the eggs outside!

raw eggs
fingernail scissors
confetti

Do this over a large bowl. With the fingernail scissors, cut a small hole at one end of the egg and a larger hole, about the size of a nickel, at the other. Clean out the egg by blowing into the small hole and allowing the insides to come out the large hole into the bowl. (Later make some scrambled eggs!) Rinse each shell carefully with water and allow to dry. Fill the egg with confetti through the large hole, then tape up the holes until ready to use. Crack them over an unsuspecting person, and watch his or her reaction.

SUREFIRE RHUBARB-STRAWBERRY CRISP

Summer is the time for this treat.

3 cups rhubarb, sliced
2 cups strawberries, whole or sliced
juice from one lemon
1 stick butter, softened
1 cup granulated sugar
1 cup flour

Preheat oven to 400°. Combine rhubarb, strawberries, and lemon juice in a 9-by-13-inch baking pan. In a medium bowl, combine the butter, sugar, and flour until crumbly and then spread over rhubarb mixture. Bake uncovered for 20 minutes or until crisp is bubbly and top browned. Serves 6.

HANDY GARDEN HINTS

🐝 With gardens burgeoning right now, many plants need to be staked—tomatoes, hollyhocks, and so on. Try tying them up with old pantyhose, which are soft enough not to cut into the stems of the plants.

🐝 If you want to capture seeds from this year's plants, zip small resealable plastic bags with tiny holes in them over the stems as the pods begin to form. (The holes will allow seeds to dry.) Remove when seeds are completely dry.

🐝 To remove the kernels on ears of corn for canning, drying, or just eating without cutting yourself, take a 4-inch piece of wood, drive a long nail into the board, and spear the ear upright onto the nail. It will be easy to cut in this position.

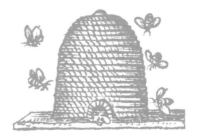

HOMEMADE GINGER ALE

This ale is very simple to make, but you've got to drink it
up after you make it—the carbonation won't last long, and
it shouldn't be sealed or it could explode.

3 tablespoons ginger root, peeled
4 quarts boiling water
1 lime
3 cups sugar
3 tablespoons cream of tartar
1 tablespoon yeast

Pound the ginger until it is a mash. Pour the boiling water over
it, and add the lime, sugar, and cream of tartar. Cover with a
cloth and let cool to lukewarm. Add yeast; let rest 6 hours.
Chill, strain, and serve. Makes 4 quarts.

ICED DELIGHTS

Spice up your ice by adding fruit, herbs, and edible flowers to the ice trays after you've filled them and before freezing. They taste great and add a visual kick to a festive occasion. Here are some fun alternatives to plain old H_2O: sprigs of rosemary, dill, lemongrass, or mint; roses, carnations, nasturtiums, lavender, or pansies; raspberries, blueberries, cucumber, lemon or lime zest.

SALT GLOW

This lotion is fabulous for exfoliating dead skin, particularly when your tan is starting to flake. Be sure not to use on your face or neck; it's too rough for that.

> 2 cups sea salt
> 7 drops of your favorite essential oil
> 1 ounce sweet almond oil

Place salt and oils in a bowl and combine well with your fingers. Stand or sit naked in an empty bathtub and rub salt mixture into your skin with your hands, starting with your feet. Massage in a circular motion. As the salts fall, pick up and reuse until you reach your neck. Then fill the tub with warm water and soak.

PLENTY OF PESTO

No book on simple pleasures would be complete without a pesto recipe. Pesto is usually made with basil, but it can also be made with cilantro or parsley or a combination. All you need is a large quantity of fresh herbs. Pesto can be frozen and lasts for several months in the freezer. If your basil is going to seed, make a large batch of pesto, minus the cheese, and freeze it. When you use it later, simply add the Parmesan.

> ¾ cup olive oil
> 1 clove garlic
> 1 tablespoon pine nuts
> ¼ teaspoon salt
> ⅓ cup grated Parmesan cheese
> 4 cups basil, cilantro, or parsley, washed

Place all the ingredients except the basil in a food processor. Process until smooth. Add the basil a little at a time, until pesto is smooth. Makes 1 cup.

ROSE WINE

Here's an old-fashioned treat. (Don't use this recipe if you spray your roses with insecticide.) Be sure to thoroughly clean the roses, and do not store wine in metal containers or stir with metal utensils; metal reacts to the acid in wine.

2 oranges
3 quarts washed and lightly packed rose petals
1 gallon boiling water
3 pounds sugar
1 package yeast
5 white peppercorns

Rind the oranges and set oranges aside. Cut up rind. Place the rose petals in a large saucepan. Pour the boiling water in and add the orange rind and sugar. Boil for 20 minutes and remove from heat and cool. Add the yeast dissolved in warm water per package instructions, the juice from the oranges, and the peppercorns. Pour into stoneware crock, cover, and let sit where temperature is between 60 and 80° for two weeks. Strain, discard petals, rinds, and peppercorns, and bottle in sterilized jars, corking lightly for about 3 months or until the wine has completed fermenting. To store wine, seal bottles with paraffin. Makes about 1 gallon.

LUSCIOUS LAVENDER

Lavender scent is very popular these days. Maybe because it is considered a romantic yet clean fragrance that is appealing to both men and women, unlike rose, for example, which is associated just with women. You can enjoy the incomparable scent of lavender, used for centuries to calm nerves, in your own home in many ways: bundles of dried lavender, lavender pillows and sachets, and lavender bath products. Lavender is also said to be good for sore, tired feet. Simply add a few drops of essential oil to a basin and place feet in water.

One incredibly easy thing to do is to buy lavender essential oil and scent your closet or chest of drawers by placing the oil on a cotton ball and rubbing it along the insides of wooden drawers and shelves. The wood will slowly release the fragrance.

PEACHES-AND-CREAM MOISTURIZER

This lotion feels fabulous on the face. In a blender or a food processor, blend one peach and enough heavy cream to create a spreadable consistency. Massage onto your skin when needed. Refrigerate unused portion. (And use up within a day or so or it will turn.)

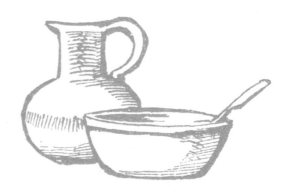

SUMMER FACIAL TONER

Here's a really easy, all-natural skin freshener, a perfect pick-me-up for hot, humid weather.

1½ cups witch hazel extract
½ cup rose water
1 tablespoon grated lime peel
1 tablespoon dried rosemary leaves
2 drops lavender oil
2 drops rosemary oil

Combine the witch hazel and rose water in a clean glass jar with a tight-fitting lid. Shake well. Add the remaining ingredients and again shake well, this time for five minutes. Store the jar in a dark, cool place, shaking five minutes a day for two weeks. At the end of that period, strain the mixture and store the remaining liquid in an airtight container, where it will last up to six weeks if refrigerated. For extra refreshment, try keeping a spritz bottle full of toner, and use it straight from the refrigerator.

WEED ARRANGING

You don't need a flower garden to create beautiful arrangements. All you need is access to a field and a bit of imagination. Wild Queen Anne's lace, bittersweet, winter cress, sea grape leaves, chive flowers, wild mustard, thistles, horsetails, and goldenrod all look wonderful in a simple vase, either all one variety or a combination. Even the simplicity of dried grasses or bare willow branches can be beautiful, while various seed pods, when dried, can make extraordinary decorations.

GASTRONOMIC TRAVEL

Looking for a way to help kids out of the end-of-summer doldrums? Try traveling without leaving home. Have your kids pick a country, then find music and food from and videos and books about that country. Look for recipes that have familiar ingredients and those that kids can make or at least help out on. You can do this activity for a day or a weekend or even for a whole week. For ideas, see *Weekends Away Without Leaving Home* by the Editors of Conari Press.

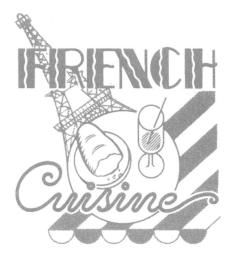

HANDMADE PIÑATA

When I moved to California, I discovered that birthday parties for kids always included a piñata. Available at Mexican markets or party supply stores, they're great for kids under ten. But you can easily construct your own (kids can help)—and you don't need to wait for a birthday. Get a very large balloon and blow it up. Cut up newspaper into ½-inch strips. Dip each strip into a bowl of undiluted laundry starch. Then wrap the strip around the balloon. Continue until the balloon is completely covered. Allow to dry completely, then paint with poster paint and cut a hole in the top (the balloon will pop; that's okay) to drop the treats in it. On either side of the big hole, cut a small hole and insert a strong cord for the hanger. Fill the balloon with candy, small gifts, nuts, and so on. (If you like, you can turn your piñata into a bird by adding construction paper head and wings, and crepe-paper feathers.) Suspend with a rope and pulley so you can raise and lower it while blindfolded adults and children take turns whacking it with a stick. When someone breaks it open, everyone scrambles for the goodies.

CHINESE ALMOND COOKIES

These are simply delicious.

½ cup whole roasted almonds
1 cup sifted all-purpose flour
½ teaspoon baking powder
¼ teaspoon salt
½ cup butter or margarine
⅓ cup granulated sugar
½ teaspoon almond extract
1 tablespoon gin, vodka, or water

Preheat oven to 350°, and grease several cookie sheets. Reserve 36 whole almonds; finely chop or grind remainder. Sift flour with baking powder and salt. Thoroughly cream butter and sugar in a large bowl. Stir in all remaining ingredients except whole almonds. Form dough into 36 balls. Place on greased cookie sheets. Press a whole almond in the center of each ball, or dot with a bit of red food coloring. Bake for 20 minutes or until lightly browned. Makes about 3 dozen.

PERSONALIZED COOKBOOKS

I try to give something meaningful to those I love as gifts and recently hit on a great idea. It all started when I began to paste recipes I clipped from magazines and newspapers in a blank book. Soon I had almost filled two books, and friends were asking me for a copy of this or that recipe. One friend asked me for so many recipes I decided to make her a cookbook for her fiftieth birthday.

I bought a beautiful blank book and divided it into sections with little tabs—appetizers, soups and salads, entrees, side dishes, and desserts. I then made chapter headings for each section, photocopied all the recipes she'd asked for or for dishes she had liked at my house, and presented the book to her. She was thrilled.

That was the end of that—or so I thought. But when my college-aged daughter started complaining that she wanted a cookbook of easy gourmet dishes for students, I knew I had to spring into action again. I hope she gets as much pleasure out of receiving it as I have been getting out of figuring out what to include.

SKIN-SOOTHER BATH

This wonderful recipe will soothe any skin condition, from heat rash to chicken pox. It's wonderful for your skin and hair, so use it even you're your skin feels fine!

> ½ cup finely ground oatmeal
> 1 cup virgin olive oil
> 2 cups aloe vera gel
> 20 drops rosemary or lavender oil

Combine the ingredients in a large bowl; stir well. Add the mixture to a warm, running bath.

THE LOVE-NOTE JAR

Here's a wonderful anniversary, holiday, birthday or Valentine's Day idea. The next special occasion, why not give your sweetheart a jar of love notes for his or her office? Simply buy an attractive jar, put a beautiful ribbon around it, and fill it with notes from your heart—"I love you because you are so gentle and kind," "I am so grateful that you are in my life"—whatever is true for you. Your honey can open the jar to be reminded of your love whenever he or she is having a bad day or feeling unappreciated.

HANDMADE TRIVETS

This is a great craft idea that is simplicity itself. Buy a plain white or terra-cotta tile from a craft store. Draw a design on it with a china-graph pencil (available at craft stores)—little kids can do handprints, which are always relished by doting parents. Then paint in your design using model paints. When completely dry, coat it with plain ceramic varnish.

CONE CAKES

This is a fun way to serve cake. You can be sure that the kids will be clamoring for more than one.

24 flat-bottomed ice cream cones
1 package (17 to 24 ounces) cake mix
muffin tins
frosting and cake decorations of your choice

Prepare the cake mix according to package directions. Spoon the batter into the cones until they are 2/3 full. Place the cones in the muffin tins and bake according to package directions for cupcakes. When cones are cool, frost and decorate. Makes 24.

ALL YOU CAN EAT

I have a friend whose family has an annual ice cream dinner one day each summer. They walk to the corner ice
cream parlor and each order a single cone, any flavor they
want. They then walk around, eating, until they're finished.
Then they return to the store and repeat the process until
they're completely satisfied. (My friend remembers that
when he turned fourteen, his record was six cones—all
strawberry.)

POTPOURRI SUPPLIES

If you are having trouble finding the ingredients to make all the wonderful potpourri recipes in this book, write to Lavender Lane, P. O. Box 7265, Citrus Heights, CA 95621 ($2 for catalogue); Rosemary House, 120 South Market Street, Mechanicsburg, PA 17055 ($2 for catalogue); or Indiana Botanic Gardens, P. O. Box 5, Hammond, IN 46325 (free catalogue).

233

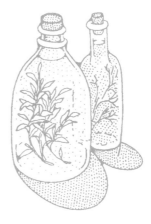

PLANT SOMETHING SPECIAL

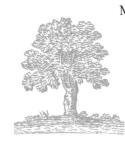

My husband and I planted a hydrangea that was on the altar at our wedding. It moves with us from house to house as a symbol of our marriage. Other people plant trees to honor loved ones who have died or to commemorate a special anniversary. And many people plant birth trees for their children. You can involve your child in helping to take care of the tree and to track its growth by tying a bit of yarn to the outmost tip of a branch each fall and see where the yarn ends up after the summer.

APLETS

Here's a recipe for a classic candy that is quite easy to make on your own.

> 2 cups applesauce
> 2 cups sugar
> 2 tablespoons unflavored gelatin
> ½ cup cold water
> 1½ cup chopped almonds
> 3 drops orange extract
> powdered sugar

Butter an 8-inch baking pan. Cook applesauce and sugar in a medium saucepan until it gets very thick. While applesauce is cooking, sprinkle the gelatin into the water and let stand. Remove applesauce from heat, and stir in gelatin. Add almonds and orange extract and stir well. Pour into baking pan. Cover and let stand on the counter overnight; do not refrigerate. The next day, cut into squares and roll in powdered sugar. Will keep up to a week or so. Serves 12.

BATH SALTS

You can feel great by making bath salts for yourself or as gifts. In a large bowl, place 3 cups Epsom salts. In a measuring cup, combine 1 tablespoon glycerin, a few drops of food coloring, and a spray of your favorite perfume. Mix well and then slowly add the liquid mixture to the Epsom salts, stirring well. Pour into decorative glass jars and tie on a ribbon bow.

WAVE AT A CHILD

H. Jackson Brown, Jr., the best-selling author of *Life's Little Instruction Book,* is great at reminding us of the simple things. I've adapted one of his ideas: today, while driving, wave to any kids you come across. If you see a schoolbus or van, great. Otherwise, wave to the kids you see in cars and notice what pleasure it gives you.

237

HEADACHE PILLOW

This is a midwestern pioneer recipe

½ ounce ground cloves
2 ounces dried lavender
2 ounces dried marjoram
2 ounces dried rose petals
2 ounces detony rose leaf
1 teaspoon orris root
2 pieces of cotton batting,
slightly smaller than a handkerchief
2 handkerchiefs
lace or ribbon, optional

Grind spices, flowers, and orris root together, either with a mortar and pestle or in a food processor. Pack the powder in between the 2 pieces of cotton. Sew together 3 sides of the 2 handkerchiefs. Place the cotton "pillow" inside and hand sew the fourth side tight enough that the contents don't leak out. Decorate with lace or ribbons, if desired. To use, lie on pillow and inhale fragrance or place over eyes.

LAVENDER BATH OIL

Here's another great way to relax

1 cup almond or grapeseed oil
½ teaspoon lavender essential oil
¼ teaspoon vitamin E oil
dried lavender sprigs
10 ounce decorative bottle with a top
ribbon and gift tag, if desired

Combine the oils in a glass container and test the scent on your skin. (You might want to add a bit more of one thing or another depending on the fragrance). Place the lavender sprigs into the bottle. Using a funnel, pour the oil into the bottle and close the top. Store in cool, dry place.

WATCH THE SUNRISE
OR SUNSET

240

It doesn't matter which you choose, although sometimes it's more fun to pick the one you usually don't see. But this time, really watch it, not as a backdrop, but, at least for the moment, as the main event.

BOW SACHETS

Here's a great present that uses lace trim scraps. You can either buy potpourri or make your own.

> 1 3-inch-wide scrap of lace trim, finished on both
> edges
> 1 3-inch-wide scrap of fine tulle
> thread to match
> potpourri
> 1-inch-wide moire ribbon

Cut a length of lace trim about 4 inches long. Place the tulle, cut to fit, on wrong side of lace and stitch along the two long and one short edges. Turn right side out and fill loosely with potpourri. Wrap the ribbon tightly around the center of the pouch, overlapping ends at back. Tuck under cut edge of ribbon and stitch it in place. Makes 1 sachet.

GILDED ANGEL

I have collected angels since before they became a craze. This angel is one of my favorites, because it is so easy to make. I made several for my house and gave some away as gifts. They look great all year round. All the supplies are available at craft stores, and there's plenty of paint left over to make more or to gild flowerpots.

> 1 terra-cotta angel of your choice
> 1 can gold spray paint
> 1 1-ounce jar white acrylic craft paint
> 1 jar clear paint thinner
> 1 small art paintbrush

Lay old newspaper down on the surface you will be working on. Spray the angel with gold paint, covering it completely, and allow it to thoroughly dry. In a paper cup or jar, make a mixture of ½ white paint and ½ paint thinner. Paint this on the angel, being careful not to create pools of paint in crevices. Immediately wipe the white paint off all the raised surfaces, leaving it untouched on the recessed surfaces to create an antique look. (You may need to rub quite hard.) Makes 1 angel.

CHILDHOOD DELIGHTS

What's your favorite food memory from childhood? Mine is my grandmother's fudge and her mustard pickles (not eaten together, thank you). I haven't had either in years. Chances are you haven't indulged in your nursery favorite either, but maybe today is the time to splurge. Do you have the recipes? If not, can you call a relative and track them down? Or try looking in *Square Meals* by Jane and Michael Stern or *Best Recipes from the Backs of Boxes, Bottles, Cans and Jars* by Ceil Dyer. Chances are your Great-Aunt Tilly's world-famous potato salad was from the Best mayonnaise jar. My grandma's "one-of-a-kind" fudge is still printed on jars of Marshmallow Fluff.

BODY BREAK

Just for today, stop thinking of your body as something that must be whipped into shape and notice what would give it pleasure. To lie down? To go for a leisurely walk? To make love? Sometimes just giving yourself permission to notice what you really desire can be an amazing way to find happiness—or at least peace of mind.

PINE POTPOURRI

This spicy concoction evokes the smell of the deep woods.

1 quart dried pine needles
1½ teaspoons essential oil such as pine or fir
1 cup chopped patchouli leaves
½ cups cinnamon sticks, broken in halves
1 tablespoon each allspice, cinnamon, cloves,
    mace, and orris root
handful of dried cranberries.

Combine the pine needles and oil in a large bowl, then add rest of ingredients. Place in a potpourri jar or glass bowl.

SEVEN-PILLOW PRINCESS (OR PRINCE) DAY

On the seven-pillow princess day, you stay in bed all day (if that appeals to you). It takes a bit of preparation, not only to find the time to goof off but also to stock up on the supplies you'll need: the books or magazines you've been longing to read, the exact food you want to eat in bed, a journal to write or draw in, polish to paint your toenails, favorite videos, and plenty of bolsters and pillows in which to luxuriate.

The point is to have a totally self-indulgent, lying-around kind of day in which you stay in bed as long as you want, doing exactly what you want, eating only what you want. (No diets allowed today!) It's a great antidote to too much running around and attending to other people's needs. Instead, you pretend you're a princess or prince and cater to your every whim. If you've got kids or a spouse, schedule one for each of you on different weekends and take turns being the baby-sitter. Believe me, it will do your heart, mind, and body good!

HEADACHE RUB

Here's an old-fashioned German cure for headaches.

> 1 quart white rose petals
> 1 quart jar, sterilized
> about 1 quart 90-proof vodka or rubbing alcohol

Pack the jar with the rose petals. Pour the vodka over and let stand, covered, for at least 24 hours. Rub mixture on forehead, temples, and back of neck.

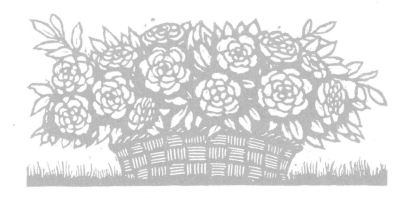

HANDMADE BANDBOXES

In the Victorian era, bandboxes were smaller versions of lady's hatboxes. You can make your own very easily by keeping your eye out for interesting shaped cardboard boxes with loose-fitting lids (so they will close when the fabric is added.) But even an old shoe box will do quite nicely, as will a heart-shaped candy box.

> 1 cardboard box with loose-fitting lid
> lightweight fabric, wallpaper,
>   or wrapping paper of your choice
> spray glue for paper, fabric glue for fabric

Place paper or fabric on the top of the lid and measure to fit, leaving 1 inch on each side to allow for overlap. Do the same for the sides of the box. Cover the side of the box by applying a light coat of appropriate glue. Fold the excess and glue to the inside and bottom of the box. Cover the top of the lid, clip the excess paper or fabric every inch or so, and then press these tabs over onto the rim and glue. Then cut paper or fabric for rim, taking care to match patterns and to conceal raw edges. Fold the top of rim down and glue to the rim of the box lid. Glue the raw edges of the rim at bottom to the inside.

BURSTS OF FLAVOR

My husband is a rabid tomato grower. After our enthusiasm for freshly picked and eaten cherry tomatoes has waned and fall has arrived, then it's time for sun-dried tomatoes. Though I have actually dried tomatoes in the sun, a much more dependable and efficient method is to dry them in an oven for five to eight hours, depending on the size of the fruit. After cleaning and splitting the tomatoes in half, I salt them lightly on oiled cookie pans and place them in a 170-degree oven. When they are dry but not crisp, I pack jars with the tomatoes and fill to the top with extra virgin olive oil (press with a spoon to make sure the air is all out, and add more oil if needed to cover tomatoes completely). We have so many sun-dried tomatoes we give lots away, but I always save some for ourselves. In the middle of winter these make the quickest and sweetest tomato paste in the world.

OLD-FASHIONED EGG CREAM

Contrary to popular belief, there are no eggs in egg creams. The name came from the fact that its taste is as rich as eggs. You really need the large fountain glasses to do this right.

2 tablespoons chocolate syrup
⅓ cup milk
⅔ cup cold seltzer water

Place the syrup in a glass. Add the milk and stir until blended. Add seltzer, stir, and serve. Makes 1 cup.

SPICY BATH SALTS

Looking for an easy-to-make natural treat for a teacher or friend? Try these fabulous bath salts. They will be greatly appreciated.

> 2 cups kosher salt
> 1 attractive glass jar with tight-fitting lid
> 2 large handfuls pine needles

Place 2 tablespoons salt evenly on the bottom of the jar. Lay 12 pine needles over the salt. Alternate salt and pine needles until the jar is full. Cover and place in a cool dark spot for four to six weeks. Add a pretty ribbon and gift tag. Makes 1 jar.

GIFTS OF THE SPIRIT

I once came across a newsletter called *Jumpin' Jan's Flash.* The author recommended eight wonderful gifts of the spirit that can really bring happiness to you and your loved ones: the gift of listening, the gift of affection, the gift of laughter, the gift of a note of love and appreciation, the gift of a compliment, the gift of a favor, the gift of solitude, the gift of a cheerful disposition. Consider the simple pleasure of giving of yourself.

PERCHANCE TO DREAM

Are you having trouble falling asleep? Consider this natural aromatherapy remedy—a sleep potion made with, among other oils, lavender. Lavender is an adaptogen, which means that it can be stimulating or relaxing, depending on your energy needs. If you are tired, it will help you fall asleep.

In a small plastic spray bottle, combine 4 drops lavender essential oil, 3 drops orange essential oil, and 3 drops chamomile essential oil (another good sleep aid), and 5 ounces of water. Shake well. Spray sheets, pillowcases, and air in bedroom before bed.

STAINED-GLASS WINDOWS

I was amazed to discover how many of my friends didn't know about these two simple crafts for kids. Both require an ironing board, a hot iron, and wax paper. For the first, pick a variety of fall leaves. Place them artfully on a piece of waxed paper and cover with another piece of waxed paper the same size as the first. Using a hot iron, iron over the leaves so that the wax melts a bit and glues the two sheets of paper together. Hang in a window.

For the second, substitute bits of crayon shavings for the leaves. When you iron the wax paper, the hot iron will melt the shavings and the colors will run together beautifully. Hang in window. Even my four-year-old could do it—with ironing help, of course.

WARM TOWELS

Before getting into the shower, put a big, fluffy bath towel in the dryer. Let it get hot and then bring it into the bathroom with you when you take a shower. Better yet, get someone else to hand it to you directly from the dryer when you step out of the water.

255

BUTTERMILK BISCUITS

These are sensational right out of the oven with butter, jelly, honey—or even plain!

2 cups all-purpose flour
2 teaspoons baking powder
½ teaspoon baking soda
½ teaspoon salt
¼ cup vegetable shortening,
    butter, or margarine
¾ cup buttermilk

Preheat oven to 450°. Combine the first 4 ingredients in a medium bowl. Cut in the shortening, butter, or margarine until the mixture resembles coarse crumbs. Stir in buttermilk. With flour-covered hands, knead gently and then roll out on floured surface to ½-inch thickness. Cut with a 2 ½-inch biscuit cutter and place on a lightly greased baking sheet. Bake for 10 to 15 minutes or until golden. Makes 10.

NATURAL PLACEMATS

For your next party, use fall leaves as place cards and mats. First dip them in warm soapy water, rinse, and allow to air dry. Then press them between the leaves of a heavy book and allow to dry for at least a week. When you remove the leaves, handle carefully because they can tear easily. Using a gold marker, carefully write the name of each person on a leaf and place on table. Create a bed of leaves at each place for a placemat. The day before, wash the leaves as described above and arrange artfully on the table.

MAKE A LOVE BOUQUET

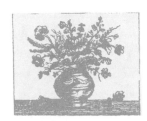

So many of us live far away from those we love. This is a simple pleasure adapted from *The Couple's Comfort Book* to bring those folks closer to you. Make a list of those who have been most important to you in your life. Then ask yourself, if he or she were a flower, what would they be? Then go to a florist and make a celebration bouquet out of all the flowers that represent your loved ones.

HERBAL BATHS

Many stores and catalogues offer wonderful "tub teas," collections of herbs packed in oversized tea bags to drop in the bathtub while it fills. If you are feeling ambitious, you can even make your own. Simply tie a few bags of an herbal tea you like to the tap. Or fill a tea infusion ball with herbs or tie up herbs in a double thickness of cheesecloth. You can even use the foot of a clean nylon stocking. Afterward, you can let the bag dry (be careful where it drips) and use it for a few more baths. Alternatively, pour a pint of boiling water over dried or fresh herbs, steep for 10 minutes, then strain into the tub. A variety of herbs are available at stores specializing in natural foods and remedies. Here are some traditional combinations. For a relaxing bath, combine chamomile, jasmine, and hops. For a stimulating bath, use marigold, lavender, bay, mint, rosemary, and thyme. For a healing bath, try calendula, comfrey, and spearmint.

SIMPLE POST-WORK PAMPERING

There are many ways to pamper yourself when you get home from work. One very simple one is to change out of work clothes and anoint yourself with an essential oil. One of our favorites is a combination we call "vamber." Pour equal parts of amber and vanilla essential oils into a vial. Shake well. The result is a uniquely rich and sensual combination that is both comforting and sexy—perfect for the evening.

DECLARE
A WATCHLESS DAY

Set aside a totally unscheduled day, with nothing to do, no
one to attend to. Take off your watch. Then follow your
own rhythm throughout the day, doing exactly what you
want, when you want.

261

THE PERFECT CUP OF TEA

Fill the kettle with fresh cold water. Bring to a roiling boil. Scald teapot with hot water. Place 1 rounded teaspoon of loose tea per cup into an infuser inside the pot (or one tea bag per cup). Pour boiling water into teapot. Let steep for three minutes. Remove tea infuser and serve.

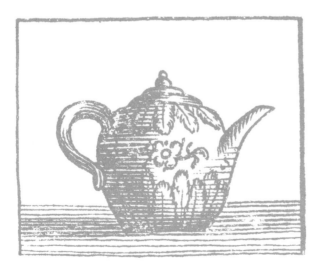

TRADING PLEASURE

Start a bulb-and-seed exchange with friends. When you are harvesting in the fall—dividing bulbs and drying out seeds for next year—try trading with friends for a no-cost way to increase the variety in your garden. We started doing this years ago when we found out the hard way that a packet of zucchini seeds was far too many for two people. We divided them up among our friends around the country, and that got the ball rolling.

To send bulbs, place them in a paper bag and then in a box. To collect seeds, shake the flower heads over an empty glass jar. To send seeds, take a small piece of paper and make a little envelope out of it by folding it in half. Take each side and fold in about ½ inch toward middle. Tape those two sides, place the seeds inside the opening at the top and then fold top down and tape again. Write on the outside what is inside, and mail in a padded envelope. A sweet surprise for family or friends.

ONION AND GARLIC BRAIDS

I love to grow onions and garlic just so that I can braid them into garlands and give them as presents. All you have to do in preparation is to leave on the long tops when you harvest your crop. Making these garlands is just like braiding hair. Cut a piece of twine as long as you want your braid to be and lay it on a table. Line up the onions or garlic in a row on the twine with the leaves all facing toward you, each onion or garlic bulb slightly overlapping the one before. Starting with the one at the top of the line, separate the leaves into three sections, incorporating the twine into one of the sections, and braid. When you are about half way down the length of the first bulb's leaves, begin to incorporate the second bulb's leaves so that the bulb sits on top of the previous braid. Continue until you reach the end of the bulbs. Dry in the sun for 3 to 5 days, and then they are ready for hanging as decorations—and to use. Simply snip off the last one on the braid as needed.

STEAMING TEA FACIAL

1 chamomile tea bag
1 peppermint tea bag
3 cups boiling water

Place the tea bags in a large, wide-mouthed bowl or pot. Add boiling water, and allow to cool for 2 minutes. Place a clean towel over your head and the bowl (keep your face at least eight inches away from the surface of the water), and steam for 10 minutes.

GO OUT ON A DATE
WITH YOURSELF

266

What do you love to do that you haven't done in a long time? Ride horseback? See a double feature? Get a massage? Make a date with yourself to do it.

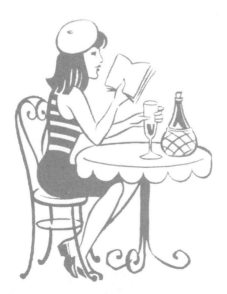

PLAYING FUN

My group of friends always holds an annual board game tournament some time in the fall. We arrive early, around 5:00 P.M., game boards in hand, have a potluck supper, and then commence playing. The more the merrier, because then there can be a game of Risk going on in one room, while Pictionary is being played in another and Dictionary in yet another. People decide what they want to play and as their game finishes, they roam around looking to join another group or to start a new game. The gaming continues until the wee hours of the morning.

SLEEPY-TIME POTPOURRI

For help with sleeping, try this potpourri in your bedroom. The lavender is said to dispel melancholy, the rosemary alleviates nightmares, and the chamomile and marjoram act as a soporific.

2 cups lavender flowers
2 cups rosemary (flowers and leaves)
1 cup chamomile flowers
2 tablespoons marjoram
2 teaspoons aniseed
2 teaspoons orris root
5 drops bergamot oil

Mix all ingredients together and place in a favorite bowl.

HOMEMADE MINT LIP BALM

The microwave makes this a snap.

1 pound jar petroleum jelly
1 microwave-safe quart container
2 tablespoons dried mint
1 ounce shredded beeswax (available at craft stores)
piece of cheesecloth
1 quart container with spout
1 ounce aloe vera
20 drops liquid vitamin E
2 tablespoons witch hazel
tiny plastic containers with lids
    (available at hardware or craft stores)

Take the petroleum jelly out of its jar and place in a microwave-safe quart container. Set the microwave on 50 percent power and heat until the jelly is soft. Put the mint and the beeswax into the jelly and heat for one minute. Stir the jelly, then heat again for another minute. (Note: stir with a nonmetal spoon so as to not flavor the liquid.) Repeat until completely melted. Take the cheesecloth and fold it in half. Strain the beeswax-petroleum jelly mixture through the cheesecloth into the quart container with spout. Discard cheesecloth. Stir in the remaining ingredients and pour into containers. Fills several containers, depending on size.

DE-STRESSING TIME WITH KIDS

The time you spend with your children may never resemble those cozy moments in TV commercials. But a few strategies may increase the pleasure. Are mornings a nightmare? Create a half hour in the evening to make lunches, collect books and other items for school, and choose clothes for the next day. Is homework a continual struggle? Help your children set up a study area. It will pay off to buy them "office" supplies, including dictionaries and other reference books. Plan to read, pay bills, and do your own office "homework" at the same time. Children won't feel that you're enjoying TV while they're struggling with algebra.

To streamline dinnertime, one woman with teenage children assigned each of them one evening a week to plan the menu and prepare the meal. Whatever the results, at least it spares you from cooking. Is bedtime an agonizing series of delays? Settle on a time for children to be in bed, then let them read for as long as they like. They may stay awake later than you'd like at first, but at least they're in bed. And they should settle into getting the amount of sleep they need.

270

HANDMADE BOOKMARKS

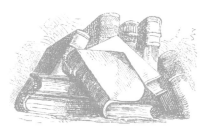

For an elegant gift, try making bookmarks out of ribbons and beads. Choose a pretty ribbon that's at least an inch wide; velvet and tapestry styles are nice. Trim the top with pinking shears to keep it from unraveling. Fold up the end of the ribbon to make a point. Tack the ends together with a couple of secure stitches in a matching thread. Sew a bead or charm onto the end of the point to weight the bookmark and add a pretty accent.

ROSE POTPOURRI

This is a real treat for rose lovers.

½ teaspoon rose essential oil
1½ tablespoons orris root (available at herb
    stores and from catalogues)
2 cups dried rose petals
2 cups dried rose geranium leaves

Combine the oil and orris root and let the mixture sit for a few days. Add to the flowers and leaves and stir well. Keep it in covered container until ready to use. Makes 4 cups.

BEAUTIFUL BOUTEILLE

This is a woven lavender wand (*bouteille* means "bottle" in French) used as a sachet to scent closets and underwear drawers. You can make an elaborate one woven like a basket, but I prefer the simplest kind possible.

273

> 40 long stalks of freshly cut lavender,
>   picked at the height of bloom
> twine or raffia
> beautiful ribbon, optional

Gather the stalks together into one big bunch. Remove any side shoots and tie together tightly just under the flowers with the twine or raffia. Bend down all the stalks evenly over the lavender blossoms and tie with twine again. Even off the ends with scissors. If you like, you can use a decorative ribbon at the end. To release the scent, simply squeeze the bouteille.

PEANUT BRITTLE

If you like peanut brittle, you must make your own!

¼ cup water

1 cup sugar

¼ teaspoon cream of tartar

½ cup light corn syrup

1½ cups roasted, unsalted peanuts

1 tablespoon peanut butter

½ teaspoon salt

½ teaspoon baking soda

Grease a large cookie sheet. In a large saucepan, bring the water to a boil and add the sugar and cream of tartar. Stir until sugar is dissolved. Stir in the corn syrup, place a candy thermometer in the pan, and cook over medium-high heat until temperature reaches 350°. Remove from heat and stir in remaining ingredients. Pour onto prepared sheet. Let cool completely, then break into pieces. You can store in an airtight container for up to 1 week. Makes about 1 pound.

"GET-IN-THE-MOOD" BATH

Here's an aromatherapy bath to inspire sensuality and enhance sexual vitality. For added fun, take it with your love partner. Run a warm bath and when tub is nearly full, light some candles, turn off the lights, and add 15 drops cardamom oil, 10 drops ylang-ylang oil, and 10 drops patchouli oil. Relax into the water and surrender to the sensations.

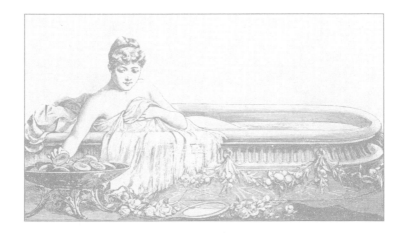

NATURAL NUANCES

The next time you host a party, lend a special touch to your table with unique and easy place cards. For inspiration, look to the great outdoors! Collect small pinecones, berry clusters, crab apples, pretty leaves, or other natural ornaments. Create a card for each guest, and use a pretty ribbon or piece of raffia to attach the cards to your natural treasures. Place one at each setting.

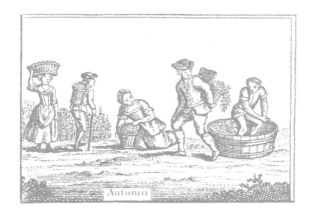

FALL WINDOW SWAG

Preserving leaves with glycerin helps them hold their color and suppleness. To preserve, mix 4 cups of glycerin into 1 gallon of water in a bucket. Take 8 to 10 cut branches with beautiful leaves, smash the stems with a hammer, and place them in the bucket. Store in a dark, dry place for 5 days until the branches have absorbed the liquid.

To make the swag, take 1½ yards of armature wire (available at craft stores). Using floral wire, attach clusters of 5 to 7 preserved leaves to the wire base. Suspend from cup hooks placed at the top of a window frame.

GIVE YOUR PLANTS
A CUP OF TEA

278

Don't throw leftover herbal tea away—use it to water your houseplants. But be sure it is caffeine free; plants like tea as long as it is "unleaded."

PINECONE BIRD FEEDER

This makes a great gift to the birds.

2 large pinecones
twine or red ribbon
hot-glue gun
½ cup peanut butter
1 15-ounce package of bird seed
two bowls, one medium, one large
two mixing spoons
small screw hooks (optional)

Hot-glue the twine or ribbon directly to the stems of the pinecones. Put the peanut butter into the medium bowl and the bird seed into the large bowl. Place a cone into the peanut butter and roll it around, pushing the peanut butter onto the cone with a mixing spoon. When it is well covered, transfer to the bird seed. Roll around, pressing the seed into the cone with the second spoon until well covered. Hang from a tree limb. Makes 2.

HOMEMADE INFUSED VINEGARS

280

Before the herbs in your garden die back, why not use them in homemade vinegars? Packaged in pretty bottles, these vinegars make a unique gift. Pick and wash the herbs to be used (long sprigs of basil, rosemary, thyme, sage, or a combination all work well and look beautiful in the bottles). Dried herbs will not work as well. The rule of thumb is 1 cup of fresh herbs per quart of vinegar. Dry herbs well on paper towels. Pack them into clean bottles or jars with lids or corks and fill with white wine vinegar that has been heated to a pre-boil. Cork or cap. Stand the jars on a sunny windowsill for about two weeks (four weeks if not very sunny). The warmth of the sun will infuse the vinegar with the herbs. Taste test; if it doesn't seem flavorful enough, strain the vinegar and add more herbs. Label and decorate the jars with a beautiful ribbon and store at room temperature. For a more lively infusion, try chile garlic vinegar: as many dried whole red chilies as will fit in your bottle, a tablespoon slightly crushed whole peppercorns, and five slightly crushed garlic cloves.

CANDLE MAGIC

An easy way to make the house cozy in fall is to use a lot of candles—in the bedroom, living room, dining room, even in the bathroom. They give a nice glow to a dark winter evening and, if scented, also add a soothing fragrance. The nice big pillar candles can get pretty expensive, but you can cut down on cost and customize your own scent by buying inexpensive, unscented votives, pillars, or tea lights at any drugstore, Pier 1, or Cost Plus. At home, anoint the candle top with a few drops of your favorite essential oil—rose, bayberry, and vanilla are nice—or use your favorite combination for a customized and affordable scented candle.

You can also decorate candles with herbs and ribbons. Use large, slow-burning candles and attach small sprigs or herbs by using a richly colored ribbon. Be sure to always place candles on fireproof saucers, and never leave them unattended! And if you want to go a step further, catalogues such as Hearthsong (800-432-6314) offer candle- and scent-making kits.

COZY UP

No hot water bottle or heating pad handy? Try moistening a thick hand towel or a modest-sized bath towel, folding it, then heating it in a microwave oven for about 1 minute and 30 seconds. Check to make sure it's not too hot, then press this "moist-heat" pad on aching muscles. When it cools down, reheat for about 30 seconds. Use a face towel for smaller aches.

Here's a dry version. Take a clean, heavyweight sock such as a cotton tube sock. Fill halfway with 4 to 5 cups of raw rice. Tie a knot in the top of the sock or wrap string around it and tie firmly. Warm in the microwave for 30 seconds at a time, until it's the right temperature. This heating pad will fit against sore muscles, especially sore necks. Take care not to get it wet.

HOMEMADE ORANGE OR LEMON PEEL

This is a nineteenth-century confection that makes a great housewarming gift.

2 quarts plus 1 cup bottled water (not tap water)	rind from 10 navel oranges or 15 lemons, halved or quartered
2 tablespoons kosher salt	4 cups granulated sugar
superfine sugar	

Combine 1 quart of water with the salt in a medium saucepan and bring to a boil. Boil for 5 minutes and set aside. When cool, pour into a large jar, add the rinds, cover and store in refrigerator for 6 days. Pour the brine into a kettle and bring to a boil. Reduce heat, add rinds, and poach for 10 minutes. Drain rinds thoroughly in a strainer and discard liquid. Combine 1 quart of water and 2 cups sugar. Bring to a boil, add rinds, and boil for 30 minutes or until peel starts to look clear around the edges. Drain rinds in colander. Cut rinds into strips. Combine remaining 1 cup water and 2 cups sugar. Bring to a boil and add rinds. Boil gently until syrup candies on the strips. Remove the strips with a slotted spoon and spread them to dry on racks. Drying time will vary depending on weather but usually takes a day. When strips are dry, dust lightly with superfine sugar and store in airtight containers. Makes 1 pound.

LOVE BATH

So named because I love to use this herbal combination.

1 cup dried lavender
1 cup dried rosemary
1 cup dried rose petals
½ cup dried lovage
½ cup dried lemon verbena
¼ cup each dried thyme,
   mint, sage, and orris root
muslin

Mix all dried herbs together and store in a covered container. When you want to take a bath, place ¼ cup of herbal mix in the center of an 8-inch square of muslin and tie tightly with a piece of string. Boil this ball in 1 quart of water for 10 minutes. Draw a warm bath, pour in the herbal water, and use the ball to scrub your body. Makes 16 bath balls.

ROSY HEART

This is a lovely homemade present from the heart.

2 dozen dried roses

2 feet 16-gauge wire (available at craft or hardware stores)

hot-glue gun

7 feet ½-inch-wide white or gold ribbon

Cut the rosebuds from the stems. Set aside. Take the wire and make a hook at each end. Bend it into a heart shape and hook the ends together at the bottom. Hot-glue one end of the ribbon to the center of the heart and wrap the ribbon all the way around the heart. When you reach the beginning, hot-glue the ribbon again to the center. With the excess, create a loop by tying the ribbon end to the heart center. With the heart flat on a table, hot-glue the rosebuds to the ribbon-covered wire. Hang in closet as a scenter or in a room as a decoration.

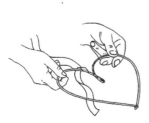
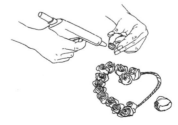

BE A JOHNNY TULIP BULB

286

Plant a few bulbs in some public place: the median strip outside your office, the corner of the park down the street, the edge of the office parking lot. You'll have fun now thinking of next spring when they suddenly burst into color.

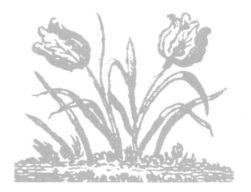

SPICED RED WINE

This concoction is a bit different from mulled wine because it is served at room temperature. You must start at least 3 weeks in advance of when you want to serve it. It's great for Thanksgiving or Christmas.

1 orange, peeled and sliced (keep the rind)
½ lemon, sliced
1 vanilla bean
6 whole cloves
1 750-ml. bottle dry red wine
½ cup framboise eau-de-vie (clear raspberry brandy) or other brandy
6 tablespoons sugar

Combine sliced orange and lemon, orange rind, vanilla bean, and cloves in large glass jar. Pour wine over. Cover and place in cool dark area for 2 weeks. Strain wine through several layers of cheesecloth into 4-cup measuring cup. Discard solids. Add framboise and sugar to wine; stir until sugar dissolves. Pour mixture into wine bottle or decorative bottle. Cork and place in cool dark area for at least 1 week. Can be made 6 weeks ahead. Store in cool dark area. Makes about 1 750-ml. bottle.

PUMPKIN BREAD

Here's a wonderful fall bread.

3 cups sugar

1 cup salad oil

4 eggs, beaten

1 16-ounce can pumpkin

3½ cups sifted flour

2 teaspoons baking soda

2 teaspoons salt

1 teaspoon baking powder

1 teaspoon nutmeg

1 teaspoon allspice

1 teaspoon cinnamon

½ teaspoon ground cloves

⅔ cup water

Generously grease and flour two 9-by-5-inch loaf pans. Pre-heat oven to 350°. Cream sugar and oil in a large bowl. Add eggs and pumpkin; mix well. Sift together flour, baking soda, salt, baking powder, nutmeg, allspice, cinnamon, and cloves. Add to pumpkin mixture alternately with water. Mix well after each addition. Pour into two loaf pans. Bake for 1½ hours, until loaves test done. Let stand for 10 minutes. Remove from pans to cool. Makes 2 loaves.

KEEPING HERBS FRESH

Fresh herbs from the grocery store are pricey, and keeping them fresh for more than a day or two can be a real struggle. If you follow a few simple tips, however, you can greatly expand their life. The trick is to treat them as you would cut flowers.

First, untie and immerse in cool water; don't run under the faucet, which can damage tender leaves. Pick through and discard any rotting stems or leaves. Shake herbs dry gently; never use a salad spinner, which is too rough. Place the bunch stems down in a vase or canning jar that allows the leaves to stay above the rim. With basil, just store on your counter top; it will keep up to a month and may even sprout roots. With all other fresh herbs, loosely cover with a plastic bag and stick in the refrigerator. Change water every few days. Chervil, chives, dill, thyme, and watercress will keep up to a week like this; cilantro and tarragon, two weeks; and parsley as long as three weeks.

SPIRITED
HALLOWEEN DECORATIONS

꙳ Cut inexpensive white tissue paper into free-form ghost and goblin shapes, then use double-stick tape to display them in your windows. Have ghoulish faces peeking in from corners or silly ones popping up over the edges. You can even put these on mirrors in your house.

꙳ Place dry ice in a large container with a bit of water to simulate a witches' brew. Be sure to keep out of reach of kids; it burns!

꙳ Hang a string of lights with orange and black bulbs.

CARAMEL CORN

This snack comes in handy when you want to host a home movie night.

⅓ cup honey
¾ cup brown sugar
2 tablespoons butter or margarine
1 cup peanuts
3 quarts popped corn

Preheat oven to 350°. In a medium saucepan, heat the honey, brown sugar, and butter or margarine until melted. On a large baking sheet, combine the peanuts and popcorn and spread in one layer. Pour the sugar mixture on top. Bake until crisp, about 10 to 15 minutes. Serves 4 to 6.

GHOULISH FUN

Make facial-tissue ghosts this Halloween. First wad up a piece of tissue or paper into a ball a little smaller than the size of a golf ball—this will serve as the ghost's head. Then put the ball in the center of another tissue and gently twist or gather the tissue around the head. White thread works well to secure the neck. Use a black felt-tip marker to draw a face—be careful, because the tissue will really soak up the ink, so err on the spare side when drawing. Then tie a piece of thread around the head and hang your ghost from the ceiling or doorway. It's really fun to make a whole bunch of these for party decorations or even to do up a bunch of blank-faced ones and let your guests draw on the expressions.

PERFECT MASHED POTATOES

High on the list of universal comfort foods is potatoes. And what could be more basic than good old mashed potatoes? This recipe comes from Jane and Michael Stern's *Square Meals*. The authors claim to have found the way to make perfect mashed potatoes. See what you think.

> 2 pounds medium potatoes, peeled and halved
> ½ cup milk
> ¼ cup heavy cream
> 3 tablespoons butter
> salt and pepper to taste

Boil potatoes in rapidly boiling salted water until they pierce easily with a fork. Drain and return potatoes to pot, and reheat until all moisture is evaporated. Transfer to mixing bowl. Mash well. Combine milk and cream in a small bowl and pour into potatoes while continuing to mash. Add butter, salt, and pepper to taste. Serve immediately. Serves 4 to 6.

HOMEMADE CANDLES

If you want to make your own candles, catalogues such as Hearthsong (800-432-6314) have kits. Or you can try the old standard we used to make in grade school. It's easy, but be careful—paraffin must be heated over low heat or it can explode. Never put it directly on the stove—only over a water bath.

block of paraffin
  (to equal 1 quart)
crayon bits for coloring
1 half-gallon coffee can
1 wick

1 pencil or chopstick
1 quart waxed cardboard milk
  or juice container, washed
  and with top cut off

Put the paraffin and crayon bits in the coffee can and place the can in a pan of water on the stove to create a double boiler. Melt the paraffin over low heat. Be sure to keep it over a very low flame, because paraffin explodes easily when overheated. While wax is melting, tie wick onto pencil or chopstick and place in the cardboard so that the pencil keeps the wick upright. When wax is melted, pour carefully into the milk or juice container and allow to harden completely overnight. Cut away container. Makes one pillar candle.

FRENCH ONION SOUP

What better way to get warm than with a wonderfully rich onion soup—truly a simple pleasure?

1 pound large white onions	3 fresh thyme sprigs
½ cup unsalted butter	or ¼ teaspoon dried thyme
1 cup dry white wine	Salt and freshly ground pepper
7 cups beef stock	1 2-day-old baguette
2 cups shredded Swiss or Gruyere cheese	

Cut the onions in half through the stem end, then again crosswise into thin slices. In a large saucepan over medium heat, melt the butter. Add the onions and wine and sauté, stirring frequently over medium heat, until onions are very soft and liquid is evaporated, about 15 minutes. Pour in the stock, add the thyme and salt and pepper to taste, and bring to a boil. Reduce heat to medium and simmer, stirring often until flavors are combined, about 15 minutes. Preheat the broiler. Cut the baguette into 6 slices. Ladle soup into 6 oven-proof bowls and place them on a wire rack or baking sheet. Place a bread slice on top of each bowl and top the slice with a liberal sprinkling of cheese. Broil 3 to 5 minutes, until cheese is melted and bubbly. Serve immediately. Serves 6.

HERBAL-BATH COLD REMEDY

When you start having the sniffles, try this soothing bath.

2 tablespoons dried eucalyptus
4 tablespoons dried rosemary
4 tablespoons dried lavender buds
2 tablespoons dried rosebuds

Steep the above ingredients in boiling water for 30 minutes. Strain and add the remaining liquid to a warm (not hot) bath.

FEED THE BIRDS

How wonderful to bring birds into your yard by putting out bird feeders. The best time to start is late fall, because the cold weather makes birds more anxious to find food and therefore more willing to try something new. Birds' body temperatures are on average ten degrees warmer than humans, and they need an almost constant food supply to stay alive. The cold weather slows down and kills the insects they eat, so they must find an alternate food supply.

It doesn't matter which side of the house you put the feeder on, but it should be protected from the wind. You should have a good view, but it shouldn't be so active in the room that the birds get scared off. At my parents' house, birds come when we were sitting quietly, but every time someone moved close to the window, they would scatter. A feeder on a pole in full view of the window but set back a little turned out to be the best compromise at my house. As for the food, wild birdseed mix is fine, as is cracked chick feed mixed with sunflower seeds for the seed-eating birds. Bug eaters such as woodpeckers shy away from seeds but love suet; you can buy special suet feeders at any bird or nature store.

"SCENT"SATIONAL IDEA

Rub your favorite essential oil (peach, rose, and vanilla are very nice atmospheric scents) on the lightbulbs in your bedroom and the night-light in the bathroom. The room will be infused with scent as light heats up the oil. For a higher-tech approach, you can also buy inexpensive clay lightbulbs rings that hold the oil. Good sources for the oils and for as all kinds of other yummy simple pleasures are the Body Time catalogue and stores (510-524-0360), the Body Shop catalogue and stores (800-541-2535), Bare Escentuals catalogue and stores (800-227-3990), Cost Plus stores, Earthsake stores, Green World Mercantile (415-771-5717), Red Rose catalogue and stores (800-374-5505), and Hearthsong catalogue and stores (800-432-6314).

MAKE A TOAST
TO THE BIRDS

Next time you empty your toaster tray of crumbs, instead of throwing them in the trash, sprinkle them outside your kitchen window. You and the birds will both be treated.

299

HONEY-SAGE TEA

This tea may not cure your cold or flu, but it sure will make you feel better.

2 tablespoons honey
juice of 1 lemon
1 ounce sage leaves, torn
boiling water

Place honey, lemon, and sage in a mug. Pour the water over and stir to dissolve honey. Cover and let sit for at least 5 minutes. Makes 1 mug of tea.

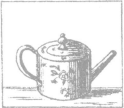

WEB TIME

Take time on a damp fall morning to observe a spider weave her web in the garden. Watch her as she moves inside the rim, patiently and methodically, reaching out her leg to catch a strand of silk from her own body, threading it to a spoke and moving on, repeating the motion again and again. It will make you marvel at the endless magic of nature. More important, twenty minutes in her company will fill you with calm.

TAKING THE WATERS

For a relaxing bath, add lavender or chamomile oil to running water. Start with ¼ teaspoon for a whole tub of water. For scents to inspire your sensuality, try ¼ teaspoon of sandalwood, ylang-ylang, or cinnamon essential oils.

For an invigorating bath, try clipping a few pieces of fresh rosemary from your garden (or buy them at the grocery store). Take a piece of cheesecloth, tulle, or fine netting and tie the rosemary up in it with a piece of twine or thread. Pound it with a mallet to release the oils. Hold the sachet under warm running water, then let it float in the bath.

LOVE DARTS

My friend Sue Patton Thoele invented Love Darts: silent blessings we send to people who are driving us crazy in some way. Rather than cursing the person silently or vociferously, Sue sends a good wish—may you be happy, for example—which if nothing else, reminds her to keep her heart open. "My favorite target," she says, "is a surly checkout person at the grocery store. I don't know how he feels about being pricked by a love dart, but I certainly feel better after sending one than I do if I grouse to myself about how rude he is." Increase your pleasure by sending love darts to anyone who annoys or frustrates you.

CLASSIC CARAMELS

Yes, the homemade ones do taste better.

1 tablespoon vegetable oil	1 cup light corn syrup
¾ cup sugar	3 tablespoons butter
1½ cups heavy cream	2 teaspoons vanilla

Line an 8-inch square baking pan with foil, extending foil over edges of pan. Coat the foil with oil. In a large, heavy saucepan, combine the sugar, cream, and corn syrup. With a wooden spoon, stir continually over medium heat until sugar is dissolved, about 5 minutes. To prevent crystallization, brush down the sides of the pot twice during the process with a pastry brush dipped in water. Place a candy thermometer in the pot and cook, stirring, over medium-high heat until the temperature reaches 250°, about half an hour. Remove from heat and add the butter and vanilla. Pour into foil-lined pan and let cool completely, at least 2 hours. Lift the caramel out of the pan with the edges of the foil. Coat a large knife with oil. Peel the foil off the caramel and cut the caramel into 8 equal strips with the oiled knife. Then cut each strip into 8 pieces. Wrap each caramel tightly in plastic wrap. Can be stored in a jar with a lid for up to 2 weeks. Makes 64.

FOR THE BIRDS

Nothing could be easier than these two treats for the birds in your life. First, make a sunflower seed wreath. Simply take a large, mature sunflower, remove the stalk from the head and cut the center from the head to form a wreath. If you want to get fancy, you can wire on other bird delights—millet, wheat, pecans. Attach a ribbon or wire hanger, and hang on a fence or tree. For the second, cut "cookies" from stale bread using cookie cutters. Poke a small hole at the top of each "ornament." Spread with peanut butter, press into a tray of birdseed. Hand from a tree using yarn threaded through hole (the birds can use the yarn in building their nests.)

CHANGE YOUR HAIRSTYLE

This is a tried-and-true simple pleasure. When feeling down, change the style or color of your hair. It really works—particularly if you end up with a great new look. I recently changed my hairstyle after having it the same for a few years, and everyone I came across in the next few months told me how great I looked. I should have done it sooner!

ELEGANT AND NATURAL DECORATIVE BALLS

You can make beautiful balls of acorns, pinecones, or cranberries for decorations or gifts. Buy some papier-mâché balls at a craft store and gather whatever items you plan to use. Using a hot-glue gun, place glue on one section of the ball, then glue pinecones, acorns, or cranberries onto the ball, as close together as possible. Continue until you've completely covered the surface. You can display these decorations on your table or a sideboard.

GREEN CHEER

A green plant is a wonderful happiness booster. One of the hardiest and easiest-to-grow plants is a sweet potato. Even if you think you have a black thumb, try this—it grows fast and it's almost impossible to kill. (OK, you do have to keep the glass full of water, but that's it.)

Get an old glass jar (a cleaned-out spaghetti sauce jar is just right) and fill it with water. Buy a sweet potato at the grocery store and poke four toothpicks in the center as if you were marking the four directions (north, south, east, and west) and place the bottom half of the sweet potato in the water. (The toothpicks will keep the whole potato from being submerged.) Place in a sunny window and wait, adding water if necessary. Soon you'll have lovely vines and big curving leaves gracing your sill.

CREATE A LOVE GALLERY

Years ago, my husband and I started putting pictures of loved ones up on a wall in our living room. They never failed to give me a lift as I walked in the door at the end of the day. We've moved several times, but our photo gallery always goes with us—hallways are a particularly good place for this. If you don't want to go to the trouble of framing photos (we buy inexpensive black frames that create a visual harmony), you can simply tack photos onto a bulletin board or attach them to the fridge with magnets—any place where they will bring a smile to your lips.

MOOD-ENHANCING SPRAY

If the dark days of late fall are dragging you down, consider this little pick-me-up—an easy-to-make rose room spray. Besides being the scent of romance, rose is said to have anti-depressant properties.

Simply combine 4 drops of rose essential oil, 2 drops of bergamot essential oil, 2 drops of lavender, and 1 cup of water. Place in small plastic spray bottle, shake well, and spray the room.

ORANGE POMANDER

Surely we all made these at some point in grade school for our mothers. They're lovely nonetheless. Take a whole orange and stud with whole cloves. Tie a string around the orange and hang in the closet where air can circulate around it. The orange will dry out, and the cloves will give a delicious fragrance to your clothes for months.

311

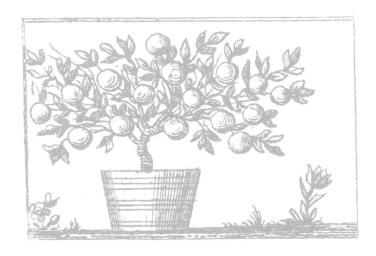

OLD-FASHIONED TAFFY PULL

Before you start, be sure to read the directions all the way through—making this does require some expertise. Above all, don't leave the little ones alone—the hot syrup can be dangerous!

1¼ cups sugar
¼ cup water
2 tablespoons rice wine vinegar
1½ teaspoons butter
1 teaspoon vanilla

In a medium saucepan over low heat, stir together the sugar, water, vinegar, and butter until sugar is dissolved. Turn heat up to medium and cook, without stirring, until the syrup reaches 265° on a candy thermometer. Pour onto a buttered platter (be careful not to be splattered by the hot syrup: hold the pouring edge away from you and pour slowly) and let cool until a dent can be made in it when pressed with a finger. Sprinkle the vanilla on top and gather the taffy into a ball. Take care in picking up the mass; it could still be very hot in the center.

When you can touch it, start pulling it with your hands to a length of about 18 inches. Then **pull** fold it back onto itself. Repeat

fold

this action until the taffy becomes a crystal ribbon. Then start twisting as well as folding and pulling. Pull until the ridges begin to hold their shape. Depending on your skill, the weather, and the cooking process, this can take between 5 and 20 minutes. Roll into long strips and cut into 1-inch pieces. Makes ½ pound.

cut

FUN FIGHT

This takes two people. Have a water, shaving cream, or food fight in the kitchen. (It's the easiest place to clean up.) If you're alone with your romantic partner, you might want to try it in the nude. If you can't stand the idea of a mess, consider a pillow fight instead. The point is to let loose!

MOUSSE IN A MINUTE

Well, maybe it will take two minutes.

1½ cups whipped topping
1 15¾ ounce can lemon or chocolate pie filling

Gently fold the whipped topping and the pie filling together in a large bowl. Spoon into dessert dishes. Serves 4.

NIGHT AT THE (HOME) MOVIES

Host a movie party for family and friends. Rent a few videos that everyone can watch, make plenty of popcorn, and offer a variety of drinks and candy treats.

COPY FALL FOLIAGE

This is a simple pleasure of the modern era—photocopying fall leaves. Just select an attractive assortment of fall foliage and place it directly onto a color copier. The copies are amazingly lifelike and can be used for decoupage projects, to cover a lampshade, to place on the front of a journal or photo album, or scattered on a table top as a fall arrangement. They will never fade, crack, or become brittle.

RED VELVET CAKE

This cake is magnificent looking and tasting!

½ cup butter, margarine, or shortening
1½ cups sugar
2 eggs
1 teaspoon vanilla
3 tablespoons cocoa
2 ounces red food coloring
2½ cups sifted cake flour
1 cup buttermilk
1 teaspoon salt
1 teaspoon baking soda
1 tablespoon white vinegar

Preheat oven to 350°. Cream shortening and sugar until smooth. Add eggs and vanilla. Beat well. In a separate bowl, blend cocoa and food coloring; add to sugar mixture. Add flour, buttermilk, and salt alternatively. Mix soda and vinegar in cup and add to batter. Bake in two greased and floured 9-inch cake pans for 30 to 35 minutes or until a toothpick inserted in the center comes out clean. Let cool before frosting.

KING OR QUEEN
FOR AN HOUR

Here's a wonderful idea for any two family members, but especially a couple, from Jennifer Louden's *The Couple's Comfort Book*.

> Flip a coin to see who will go first. The partner who wins the coin toss rules for the next hour. Agree ahead of time that no request is out of bounds; the person of the hour is to be treated to whatever he or she wishes. When the hour is up (use a timer), the next person is crowned for his or her hour of royalty.

HUG SOMEONE TODAY

Like with so many other positive acts, it turns out that hugging boosts our immune systems. Plus, it just plain feels good! So hug someone today, perhaps a person who seems particularly in need.

MONTICELLO WINE JELLY

This recipe is adapted from a dish served on Thomas Jefferson's table. (But you can be sure he didn't make it himself!) It can be served as a side dish or dessert. Adults only, please; this one contains alcohol.

½ cup cold water
2½ envelopes
   unflavored gelatin
2 cups grape juice
pinch of salt

¾ cup sugar
2 cups dry red wine
   such as Burgundy
juice of 3 lemons
fresh grapes for garnish

Put the water in a medium bowl and stir in the gelatin until dissolved. In a small saucepan, bring the grape juice to a bowl, then stir into the gelatin mixture. Add the salt and sugar and stir. When completely cool but not set, stir in the wine and lemon juice. Pour gelatin into 6 to 8 wine glasses (depending on size of glass) and chill until firm, at least 2 hours. When ready to serve, garnish with grapes. Serves 6 to 8.

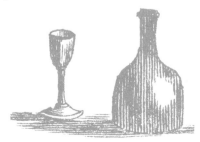

RITUAL OF APPRECIATION

You can do this any time, anywhere, but this ritual, which I call "Appreciations," is great around the Thanksgiving table. It's wonderful for bringing people closer, even those who don't know one another very well (because you can always find something to appreciate about someone, even if it is the brussel sprouts casserole he contributed to dinner). It's really effective with alienated kids who tend to hear nothing but complaints about them most of the time.

"Appreciations" works best when everyone chooses one person as the focus and then everyone else, as the spirit moves them, speaks about that person. When everyone who wants to has spoken, move on to the next person. There are four rules: remarks must be positive (no sarcasm or backhanded compliments), no one else may interject anything while someone is speaking, no one has to speak if he or she doesn't want to, and the object of the appreciations, instead of responding, just silently takes in the praise. It's surprising how difficult this last rule is—but you'll get used to it!

322

EASY THANKSGIVING DECORATIONS

🍂 Roll up your fabric napkins and tie with brown twine. Place a cinnamon stick or a leaf under the twine. Make a knot one inch from the end of the twine, and unravel the twine up to the knot.

🍂 Gather enough pinecones to have one for each person eating with you. Use them as place cards by writing each person's name on a slip of paper and tucking it into the scales of the cones.

FAVORITE FOODS

At Thanksgiving many families get very particular about their traditional foods. Take some time to make sure you are including the things that say "holiday" to you. Even when I am invited to someone else's house for Thanksgiving, I always bring the cranberry sauce, because I am so particular about how it is made. What's your Thanksgiving simple pleasure?

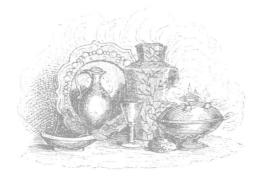

CANDIED SWEET POTATOES

Many folks swear by this tried-and-true side dish.

1 cup dark corn syrup
½ cup firmly packed dark brown sugar
2 tablespoons corn oil margarine
12 medium sweet potatoes, cooked, peeled,
   and halved lengthwise
handful miniature marshmallows, optional

Preheat oven to 350°. In a small saucepan, heat corn syrup, brown sugar, and margarine to boiling; reduce heat and simmer 5 minutes. Pour ½ cup of the syrup into a 13-by-9-by-2-inch baking dish. Arrange potatoes, overlapping if necessary, in syrup. Top with remaining syrup. Add marshmallows if using. Bake, basting often, for 20 minutes, until well glazed. Makes 12 servings.

THANKSGIVING CENTERPIECE

Here's an idea that is so simple you won't believe how good the end result will look. This Thanksgiving, why not decorate your tabletop with a collection of gourds and squashes? In the center of your arrangement, place the "Mayflower." To make it, find a large gourd in the shape of a boat and decorate with skewer masts and paper cutout sails. Finish off by scattering fall leaves, pinecones, and acorns among the squashes.

CRANBERRY APPLE WALDORF

Here is another holiday standard.

3 envelopes unflavored gelatin	3½ cups cranberry juice cocktail
⅓ cup sugar	1 cup chopped apple
1 cup boiling water	½ cup chopped celery
	⅓ cup chopped walnuts

In a large bowl, mix gelatin and sugar; add boiling water and stir until gelatin is completely dissolved. Add cranberry juice; chill until mixture has the consistency of unbeaten egg whites. Fold in apple, celery, and walnuts; pour into 8- or 9-inch square pan and chill until firm. To serve, cut into squares. Makes about 8 servings.

327

THANKSGIVING CONNECTIONS

🕊 Say thanks. If you have trouble knowing what to say, you might want to pick up a copy of *A Grateful Heart: Daily Blessings for the Evening Meal from Buddha to The Beatles* by M. J. Ryan. Or hold hands and go around in a circle, saying one after another: "May the love that is in my heart pass from my hand to yours."

🕊 Go around the table, with each person naming one thing they are particularly grateful for this year.

🕊 Ask everyone to speak of who or what has been the greatest teacher in their life and why.

🕊 Tell a story of how you celebrated Thanksgiving when you were a child.

🕊 Invite the new person at the office who just relocated, or someone you know will be alone, to your home for Thanksgiving dinner and include him or her in your traditions.

CRANBERRY PUNCH

This festive warm drink is nonalcoholic, so it can be enjoyed by everyone.

6 cups cranberry juice

2 cups lemonade

½ teaspoon each ground cinnamon, cloves, and allspice

1 cup sugar

2 lemons, thickly sliced

24 whole cloves

Simmer all ingredients, except lemons and whole cloves, for 15 minutes. While the punch is cooking, stud the lemons with the cloves. When punch is ready, place in punch bowl or Crock-Pot and float the lemons on top. Serves 12.

SAUL'S LATKES

This recipe is courtesy of Saul's Deli in Berkeley, California, the best Jewish deli west of New York City.

2 large peeled russet potatoes
1 large egg
1 tablespoon flour
   or matzo meal

salt and pepper to taste
peanut oil
applesauce and sour cream,
   optional

Using the largest holes of a grater, or the grater on the Cuisinart, grate potatoes into a large bowl. Sprinkle flour or matzo meal over potatoes, add salt and pepper, and mix well with a fork. Break the egg into the potatoes and mix with a fork. In a cast-iron skillet, pour enough peanut oil to make a ⅓-inch layer and heat very slowly—don't let the oil smoke. When oil is hot, spoon latke mix into oil and flatten with a spatula. Fry till golden brown, about 4 minutes, then flip over, reduce heat, and fry the other side, about 3 minutes. Drain onto paper towels and serve with applesauce and sour cream, if desired. Serves 2.

SPICING UP
THE FLAMES

The next time you light a fire, sprinkle a few drops of frankincense, cedarwood, or pine essential oil onto a log before lighting it, and you will enjoy an even more fragrant fire.

CANDLE SYMBOLISM

Candles are wonderful, especially as the dark creeps in earlier and earlier. If you would like to be intentional about the candles you use, consider the symbolism of various colors:

WHITE: spiritual truth and household purification

GREEN: healing, prosperity, and luck

RED: physical health and vigor

YELLOW: charm and confidence

SIMPLE NAPKIN RINGS

Here's a project kids can help with. You can modify these rings for any holiday or occasion by using different wrapping papers: red, white, and blue for the Fourth of July. Stars of David for Hanukkah, balloons for birthdays, and so on.

> 2 empty toilet paper rolls
> utility knife or Exacto knife
> scissors
> glue
> festive wrapping paper

Carefully cut the toilet paper rolls into 1½-inch sections with the utility knife. (Measure from an end and make four marks around the roll as a guide.) You will now have six rings. Take the wrapping paper and cut it into 6 4-by-6-inch rectangles. Put glue on the back of the paper and wrap one rectangle around each ring, tucking and overlapping on the inside. Makes 6 napkin rings.

OLD-FASHIONED GIFTS

The Vermont Country Store in Weston concentrates on items that are no longer available but were once popular and useful. This kind of merchandise fills a need, not because of nostalgia but because it worked and kept on working. In the store's catalogue you'll find nightshirts, all-cotton sheets, chenille bedspreads, badger shaving brushes, thick, hotel-quality bath towels, garden weeding tools, and a variety of old-fashioned soaps and health remedies. For a catalogue, call 802-362-2400.

The Cumberland General Store in Crossville, Tennessee, is a time machine transporting you back a hundred years. Its catalogue includes old-style kitchenware such as soapstone griddles and coffee percolators, a handmade Amish rocking chair, hard-to-find cakes of Bon Ami cleanser, toy wooden tops and wire puzzles, kits for recaning chairs, dulcimers—and even a ready-to-assemble windmill. Call 800-334-4640. And L. L. Bean of Freeport, Maine, may have edged into the mainstream, but the catalogue is still a good place to shop for hand-sewn moccasins, warm flannel sheets, and Adirondack chairs. Call 800-221-4221.

YUMMY GINGERBREAD

This old-fashioned gingerbread recipe dates back to colonial New England and is ideal for creating holiday "gingerbread people."

5 cups flour
3 cups sugar
1½ teaspoons baking soda
2 tablespoons ground ginger
1 pound butter, softened
3 eggs
1½ cups milk

Preheat oven to 375°. Sift together flour, sugar, baking soda, and ginger. Gradually combine with butter (mixture will feel coarse and crumbly). In a separate bowl, combine the eggs and milk, then add to the flour mixture, stirring until well blended. With a floured rolling pin, roll the dough out thinly onto a large baking sheet. With a cookie cutter, cut out shapes and place on a greased cookie sheet. Bake 5 to 10 minutes, or until brown.

THE KINDNESS BOX

During the weeks leading up to the holidays, we keep a kindness box. We wrap up a shoebox like a present and cut a slot in the top. Then we put the box and a pencil and some paper under the tree. When someone in the family notices someone doing something kind, we write the act down on a piece of paper and put it in the box. (Young children could draw a picture or tell Mom what they saw and ask her to write it down.) On Christmas Eve, along with reading a beautiful picture book of the Christmas story, we open the box and read all the notes.

EXPERIENCING GREAT HOLIDAYS

When you think of the six-week period between Thanksgiving and the first of the year, do you look forward to the time with eager anticipation or a sense of dread? For so many of us, the holidays, which should be filled with opportunities for pleasure—a sense of togetherness, a chance to give, a chance to be grateful—are instead occasions for fights, disappointment, overspending, and fatigue.

Today, just take a moment to figure out why the holidays are not pleasurable for you. Do you or those around you have unrealistic expectations that you run around trying to fulfill? Do you overspend? Do the holidays bring up feelings of loneliness? Do you have trouble getting along with the relatives that you will spend time with? Today all you have to do is to identify where the holidays get derailed for you and to make a commitment to finding ways to increase your holiday pleasure.

FLOWERPOT CANDLES

The scent I've suggested is for Christmas, but feel free to substitute your own favorite essential oils. This recipe is for one candle but can be multiplied for more.

1 3-inch clay flowerpot	1 ounce beeswax
small piece of	1 ounce paraffin wax
self-hardening clay	15 drops cinnamon
1 6-inch candlewick	essential oil
1 small stick at least	15 drops mandarin orange
5 inches long	essential oil

Plug the hole in the bottom of the pot with the clay and let harden. Attach one end of the wick to the stick. Lay the stick on top of the pot with the wick hanging down in the center of the pot. In a double boiler, melt the beeswax and add the paraffin. When melted, remove from heat and let cool slightly. Add the essential oils and mix thoroughly. Pour the wax slowly into the pot, reserving a little bit. Fill to within ¼ inch of top. If a hollow forms around the wick as the wax cools, pour more wax into hollow. Once wax has hardened, remove stick by trimming the wick. Makes one candle.

HANDMADE SNOWFLAKES

When I was a kid, we always used to make snowflakes by folding white paper and then cutting out intricate patterns with scissors. Then we'd Scotch-tape them onto the front windows. Try it with your kids—or by yourself!

339

MAGIC REINDEER FOOD

Here's a great inexpensive gift idea for Brownie leaders, teachers, and anyone else. Or you can just make it for your kids. Fill a baggie with about 1 teaspoon of red and green glitter and ¼ cup instant oatmeal. Attach a Xeroxed picture of a reindeer and the following saying: "On Christmas Eve, sprinkle this Magic Reindeer Food on your lawn. The Magic Glitter sparkling in the moonlight and the smell of oats will guide Rudolf to your home." To make the magic food even cuter, glue a red pom-pom to the reindeer's nose. Remember to sweep up the oats after the kids have gone to bed, because they will ask the next morning why Rudolf didn't eat them.

HOT BUTTERED RUM

This drink is a true winter tradition.

1 teaspoon brown sugar
2 ounces rum
4 ounces (½ cup) hard cider
1 tablespoon butter
pinch of grated nutmeg

Combine sugar and rum in a mug or glass. Over medium heat, warm cider to a preboil, then add butter, stirring until melted. Pour into mug, and serve immediately, dusted with nutmeg. Serves 1.

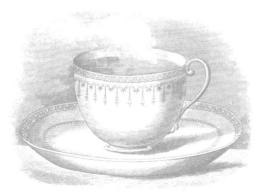

CHRISTMAS PLEDGE

Last year, my family took the Christmas pledge as described in the book *Unplug the Christmas Machine*. It goes like this:

Believing in the beauty and simplicity of Christmas, I commit myself to the following:

1. To remember those people who truly need my gifts.
2. To express my love for family and friends in more direct ways than presents.
3. To rededicate myself to the spiritual growth of my family.
4. To examine my holiday activities in light of the true spirit of Christmas.
5. To initiate one act of peacemaking within my circle of family and friends.

WEDGWOOD WASSAIL

In modern times, wassail is usually served indoors, at holiday parties. This recipe, which can be made nonalcoholic, is from the Wedgwood Inn in New Hope, Pennsylvania.

> 1 gallon apple cider
> 2 quarts cranberry juice
> 1 tablespoon whole allspice
> 2 oranges, studded with cloves
> 4 sticks cinnamon
> 2 cups rum, optional

In a 2-gallon pot, combine all ingredients and heat gently. Serve warm. Makes 24 servings.

SCENTED ORNAMENTS

Here's another wonderful and simple decorating idea. No, the ornaments are not edible!

1 4-ounce can ground cinnamon (about 1 cup)
1 tablespoon ground cloves
1 tablespoon ground nutmeg
¾ cup applesauce
2 tablespoons white glue
thread
glitter glue, fabric, or other decorating items,
   optional

In a medium bowl, combine cinnamon, cloves, and nutmeg. Add applesauce and glue; stir to combine. Work mixture with hands 2 to 3 minutes or until dough is smooth and ingredients are thoroughly mixed. Divide dough into 4 portions. Roll out each dough portion to ¼-inch thickness. Cut dough with cookie cutters. Using a toothpick, make small hole through the top of each ornament. Place cut-out ornaments on wire rack to dry. Allow several days to dry, turning ornaments over once a day. Create hangers by pushing a length of thread through the hole at the top of each one. Decorate as desired with glitter, beads, or fabric.

NATURAL STOCKINGS

Make a unique Christmas stocking for your loved ones. Simply buy a plain red stocking and a 5-inch-wide piece of rug-hooking mesh (available at needlecraft stores). Sew the mesh to the stocking and then tuck small bits of evergreen branches or colored leaves into the mesh.

CANDY CANE POTPOURRI

If you are a fan more of the scent than the taste of peppermint, consider this holiday potpourri.

4 cups dried peppermint leaves
3 cups dried pink rose petals and buds
1 cup dried hibiscus flowers
1 tablespoon whole cloves
1 tablespoon broken pieces of cinnamon sticks
2 tablespoons orris root
    (available at herbal stores and from catalogues)
20 drops rose essential oil
10 drops peppermint essential oil
1 tablespoon gum benzoin
    (available at herbal stores and from catalogues)

Combine all ingredients except gum benzoin and stir well. Add gum benzoin and stir well again. Makes 2 quarts.

PINECONE ORNAMENTS

Make sure that the size of the ribbon and the roses is proportionate to the size of the cones.

small pinecones
7-inch lengths of very narrow ribbon
dried rosebuds
glue gun

Place pinecones in a paper bag. Put into the microwave and heat for 8 to 10 minutes. (This is to kill bugs.) If you want the cones to open and this hasn't opened them, keep heating the same way at 3-minute intervals until they open. Take the ribbon, fold it in half, and hot-glue the ends to the stem end of the cone. Take a bud or two and hot-glue them on top of the ribbon ends to hide them. Repeat until all cones are done.

CAROLING IDEAS

Some of my fondest memories are about Christmas caroling in my neighborhood in the snow. To make caroling truly memorable for you, consider the following:

- Bring people together a half hour early for practice.
- Have a sheet with lyrics for everyone.
- Don't forget flashlights.
- Consider singing at a nursing home or homeless shelter.
- Finish back at your house with hot chocolate and cookies!

MISTLETOE BALL

Instead of a little sprig of mistletoe in your doorway, how about hanging a beautiful kiss-inspiring ball? It's easy to make.

> 1 6-inch-wide ball of floral foam
> chicken wire, the same size as the foam
> decorative cord or ribbon for hanging the ball
> various evergreens such as pine, holly, and hemlock
> mistletoe

Soak the floral foam in water until thoroughly wet. Wrap it in the wire and tie the ribbon or cord of desired length to the chicken wire. Insert small pieces of greens into the foam to create a pleasing circular shape. Insert mistletoe at the base of circle so it hangs lower than the rest of the greens. Hang in doorway. You know the rest!

VICTORIAN CHRISTMAS DECORATION

350

Decorate your table with sugared fruit, an old-fashioned Christmas tradition. Dip apples, pears, plums, and grapes into egg white and then roll in granulated sugar. Arrange attractively in a bowl.

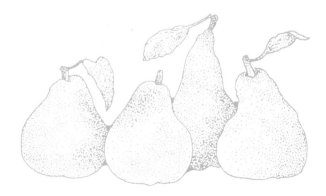

OLD-FASHIONED TOYS

Are you looking for the toys from your youth for your children or grandchildren—things like wooden Tinkertoys and Lincoln Logs, Raggedy Anns, pogo sticks, American Eagle sleds, and so forth? Well, look no further than the Back to Basics toy catalogue. For a copy, call 800-356-5360.

SIMMERING
HOLIDAY POTPOURRI

Here's a mixture you can make for holiday gifts for teachers or for open houses and other get-togethers when you want to bring a little something. Be sure to package with directions.

1 cup whole allspice	2 cups orange peel, cut into slices
1 cup star anise	2 cups rose petals
1 cup fresh ginger,	2 cups lemon verbena leaves
cut into slices	30 drops allspice oil

Combine all ingredients except allspice oil in a large container. Stir in oil 5 drops at a time until mixture is well combined. Store in airtight container or, if you want to use as gifts, package in baggies or small jars. To use, pour ⅔ cup into 2 to 3 cups of water and simmer gently on stove to release aroma. Can be reheated until scent is gone. Makes about 10 cups.

HYDRANGEA WREATH

This wreath is the height of simplicity and beauty. Buy a plain evergreen wreath (during the holidays, the Boy Scouts sell them outside my local supermarket). Take five bunches of dried hydrangea blossoms and insert them in the wreath equidistant from one another. If the stems aren't long enough to secure by themselves, attach with florist's wire. Make five simple bows that complement the hues in the hydrangeas (teal-blue moire silk is spectacular, but ivory or pink might also work). Attach a bow with florist's wire to each hydrangea bunch. Hang indoors.

TREE-TRIMMING CIDER

This cider is always a big hit at my house.

16 whole cloves
2 large apples, peeled but left whole
1 gallon apple cider
3 cinnamon sticks
ground nutmeg

Insert 8 cloves into each apple. Pour the cider into a large pot and add the apples and cinnamon sticks. Bring to a boil; then cover and reduce heat to low. Simmer for 1 hour to allow flavors to blend. Discard apples and cinnamon and ladle hot punch into mugs. Sprinkle with nutmeg and serve. Makes 16 servings.

ORANGE AND BAY GARLAND

This garland requires a bit of planning.

3 oranges
metal skewers
1 yard string
8 cinnamon sticks
100 fresh bay leaves
1 large darning needle

Make a series of vertical cuts into the oranges, but do not cut all the way through. Thread through one of the slits onto the skewers, and come out the backside through another slit. Rest the skewers across a baking pan so that the oranges are suspended over the pan. Place in a cooling oven and let sit until the orange skins have hardened. Let sit in a warm, dry place for 1 week or so to continue drying. To make the garland, tie a knotted loop at one end of the string. Tie a cinnamon stick next to the loop. Thread the darning needle onto the other end of the string and then thread 10 bay leaves by skewering them through the middle with the needle. Tie another cinnamon stick on and thread another 10 bay leaves. Thread an orange through the center. Repeat until you've used up all the materials. Makes a 30-inch garland that can be tacked to a mantle.

CELEBRATE LIGHT

On solstice night (December twenty-first), gather candles and matches and then turn off all the lights in your home. After dwelling on the dark for a few moments, light the candles and welcome the light back into the world.

356

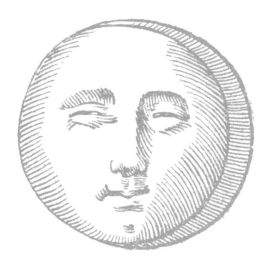

MULLED WINE

This recipe is great any time the weather turns cold.

2¾-liter bottles dry red wine
6 tablespoons sugar
8 whole cloves
4 cinnamon sticks
1 orange, sliced into rounds with peel left on
1 lemon, sliced into rounds with peel left on
1 whole nutmeg, crushed
4 tablespoons rum or cognac, optional

In a large pot over medium high heat, combine all the ingredients except rum or cognac, stirring until sugar is dissolved and the wine is hot but not boiling. Remove from heat and add the rum or cognac, if desired. Let sit for 10 minutes, then remove solids and serve. Makes 8 servings.

TRIM-TRIMMING SUGGESTIONS

Here are some ideas I've gathered from friends:

358

- Buy a small live evergreen and decorate it with popcorn and cranberry strands, which kids love to make, and when the holidays are over, plant it outside, complete with decorations.

- Decorate a live tree with tiny bouquets of dried flowers and use thin ribbon as hangers.

- Bundle cinnamon sticks together with raffia and hang them from the tree, along with bundles of small pinecones and holly twigs wired together with garden wire.

- Decorate with seashells you've collected. Starfish, sand dollars, and sea urchins can be draped on branches and tiny holes can be drilled in scallop shells so they can be hung.

- Kids also love to make paper chains.

- Tie family photos to the tree to bring loved ones who are far away closer.

- Save the little boxes that paper clips and toothpicks come in and wrap them like little presents with scraps of wrapping paper and narrow ribbon.

CITRUS ORNAMENTS

These look beautiful on the tree.

> 3 to 4 lemons, oranges, and/or limes
> gold cord
> various small dried flowers and leaves
> berries, narrow ribbon, and other decorative items
> glue gun

Cut the fruit into ¼-inch slices. Place four layers of paper towels on a microwave-safe plate and arrange the citrus slices on the paper towels. (If they don't all fit in one layer, do it in batches.) Cover with another sheet of paper towel and heat at 50 percent power for 2 minutes. Turn the slices over and place them on dry spots. Repeat until dry. (Note: If the bottom towels become too wet during this process, replace with four new sheets.) Cut the gold cord into 6-inch lengths, 1 piece for each slice. Fold cord in half and glue the ends together to the back of a citrus slice. Pick out various dried flowers and leaves, and bits of ribbon and other trim, and glue them to the front of the slice.

HOLIDAY NAPKIN RINGS

These napkin rings can do double duty as place holders if you add small tags and write each person's name on them. They are so quick you can make them just a few minutes in advance.

> 6 bendable tree twigs such as silver birch,
>   long enough to have a 3-inch circumference when bent
> floral wire
> silver or gold ribbon
> small dried red roses
> glue gun

Twist twigs into rings and fasten with floral wire. Make a small bow with the ribbon and tie onto each of the rings. Make sure that when the ring is flat on the table, the bow is also horizontal. (If necessary, carefully hot-glue the bow.) Next, hot-glue a small bunch of dried roses around the bow and over the knot to create a splash of color. Makes 6 napkin rings.

CANDY CANE
HOT CHOCOLATE

If you are a hot chocolate lover, try spicing it up with peppermint. Either melt a few peppermint candies by stirring them into the pot while you're making the hot chocolate (taste test to get the amount right), or serve the chocolate in mugs with a whole candy cane as a stirrer.

SNOWBALL SURPRISES

These are great for kids to make and to eat.

8 ounces butter or margarine, softened
¾ cup sugar
1 teaspoon vanilla
2 cups flour, sifted
8 ounces Hershey's Kisses, unwrapped
powdered sugar

Cream the butter or margarine and sugar. Add the vanilla and mix well. Add flour, combine well, and wrap in plastic and refrigerate for half an hour. Preheat oven to 350°. Take dough out of refrigerator and break into balls large enough to cover a Hershey's Kiss. Insert the Kiss, making sure it is completely covered. Bake on ungreased cookie sheet until cooked through, about 10 to 12 minutes. While still warm, sift powered sugar on top. Makes 2½ dozen.

HOPPIN' JOHN

It's said in the South that if you eat this on New Year's Day, you will have good luck all year. To make it vegetarian, simply omit the ham hocks and add a bit of soy sauce.

1½ cups dry black-eyed peas
4 cups water
1½ cups chopped onions
3 cloves garlic, chopped
½ teaspoon pepper

¼ teaspoon red pepper
1 bay leaf
8 ounces ham hocks
salt and pepper

Bring peas and water to a boil in a large saucepan. Boil two minutes and remove from heat. Let stand 1 hour. Add remaining ingredients, cover, and simmer for two hours, stirring frequently. Add more water if necessary. Remove ham hocks and bay leaf, add salt and pepper to taste. Serve over rice. Serves 4.

EIGHTEEN-CARAT EGGNOG

Only you can decide if drinking this glorious eggnog is worth the risk of consuming raw eggs. The recipe's creator has been making it for years with no ill effects—she claims the alcohol kills any potential bacteria. She also says the longer it ages, the better it tastes, and it will keep refrigerated for up to a year.

9 egg yolks
2½ cups superfine sugar
3⅓ cups (1 750-ml. bottle) bourbon
1½ cups plus 2 tablespoons light rum
1½ cups plus 2 tablespoons brandy
1 quart heavy cream
2 cups half-and-half
freshly grated nutmeg

Whisk the yolks and the sugar together by hand in a large bowl (a 13-quart one works best). Slowly stir in the bourbon, rum, brandy, cream, and half-and-half. Pour into glass jars and refrigerate, covered, for at least three days. Shake the jar very well before serving the eggnogg. Serve over ice with a sprinkle of freshly grated nutmeg. Sip slowly and enjoy! Serves 12.

OPEN HOUSE

Every New Year's afternoon, we host an open house for the entire neighborhood from 3:00 to 5:00. This tradition started when we first moved into town and didn't know anyone. We just printed up invitations on our computer, making it clear we were inviting the whole neighborhood, and stuck them under the front doors of the houses in the surrounding neighborhood. We had quite a turnout—most people work and don't know one another and were eager to meet. Once we got started, everyone wanted to do it again. It's a very low-key affair—I serve a few simple appetizers and hot mulled cider, and most folks bring something to add to the buffet table. It's a nice way to end the holiday season, and at least we all get a chance to catch up with one another once a year. Try it in your neighborhood.

365

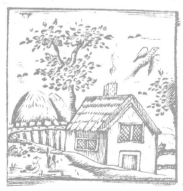

NATURE'S HANGOVER CURE

Here's something to try, if necessary (hopefully not!), on New Year's Day.

1 tablespoon finely chopped fresh ginger root
1 teaspoon grated lemon peel
2 cups water
¼ cup culinary rose water
1 drop peppermint oil

Combine the ginger root, lemon peel, and water in a covered pot and bring to a boil. Simmer 10 minutes. Strain out ginger and lemon peel pieces and cool the remaining liquid. Add rose water and oil of peppermint. Drink ½ cup at room temperature every 2 hours, along with plenty of water.

INDEX

If you enjoyed 365 *Simple Pleasures,* you might enjoy these other books from Conari Press:

Simple Pleasures
by Robert Taylor, Susannah Seton, and David Greer

Simple Pleasures of the Home by Susannah Seton

Simple Pleasures for the Holidays by Susannah Seton

Simple Pleasures of the Garden by Susannah Seton

365 Health and Happiness Boosters by M. J. Ryan

TO OUR READERS

ONARI PRESS publishes books on topics ranging from spirituality, personal growth, and relationships to women's issues, parenting, and social issues. Our mission is to publish quality books that will make a difference in people's lives—how we feel about ourselves and how we relate to one another. We value integrity, compassion, and receptivity, both in the books we publish and in the way we do business.

As a member of the community, we donate our damaged books to nonprofit organizations, dedicate a portion of our proceeds from certain books to charitable causes, and continually look for new ways to use natural resources as wisely as possible.

Our readers are our most important resource, and we value your input, suggestions, and ideas about what you would like to see published. Please feel free to contact us, to request our latest book catalog, or to be added to our mailing list.

2550 Ninth Street, Suite 101
Berkeley, California 94710-2551
800-685-9595 • 510-649-7175
fax: 510-649-7190
e-mail: conari@conari.com
www.conari.com